Praise for *The 30-Minute Vegan*:

"*The 30-Minute Vegan* is not only a culinary delight for vegetarians and vegans, it appeals to people who relish a meal that luxuriates the palate and satisfies the spirit."

—Michael Bernard Beckwith, author of
Spiritual Liberation: Fulfilling Your Soul's Potential

"Don't let a lack of time keep you from making a healthy choice! These quick, delicious recipes will see you through even the busiest mealtimes with good taste and style."

—Jennifer McCann, author of *Vegan Lunch Box* and
Vegan Lunch Box Around the World

"Mark Reinfeld and Jennifer Murray have written a classic, practical guide to preparing exquisitely tasteful, healthy vegan food that is ideal for busy folks of today. Every home will be enriched by having this book in the kitchen. It is suitable for daily meals prepared for family members, as well as special holiday celebrations."

—Arthur H. Brownstein, M.D., M.P.H., author of
Healing Back Pain Naturally and *Extraordinary Healing*

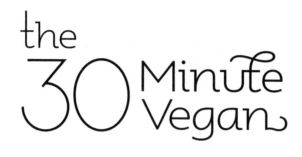

Also by Mark Reinfeld and Jennifer Murray

The Complete Idiot's Guide to Eating Raw (with Bo Rinaldi)

Also by Mark Reinfeld

Vegan Fusion World Cuisine (with Bo Rinaldi)

the
30 Minute
Vegan

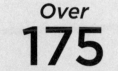

Over
175 Quick, Delicious, and Healthy
Recipes for Everyday Cooking

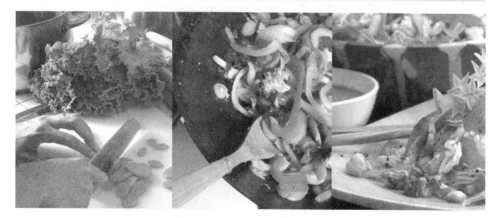

Mark Reinfeld and Jennifer Murray

Foreword by Deborah Madison

Da Capo
LIFE
LONG

DA CAPO PRESS
A Member of the Perseus Books Group

Copyright © 2009 Mark Reinfeld and
    Jennifer Murray
Foreword copyright © 2009 Deborah Madison
Photographs by: Mark Reinfeld and
    Jennifer Murray

Designed by Trish Wilkinson
Set in 11-point Minion by the Perseus
    Books Group

Cataloging-in-Publication data for this book is available from the Library of Congress.

First Da Capo Press edition 2009
ISBN: 978-0-7382-1327-9

Published by Da Capo Press
A Member of the Perseus Books Group
www.dacapopress.com

Note: The information in this book is true and complete to the best of our knowledge. This book is intended only as an informative guide for those wishing to know more about health issues. In no way is this book intended to replace, countermand, or conflict with the advice given to you by your own physician. The ultimate decision concerning care should be made between you and your doctor. We strongly recommend you follow his or her advice. Information in this book is general and is offered with no guarantees on the part of the authors or Da Capo Press. The authors and publisher disclaim all liability in connection with the use of this book. The names and identifying details of people associated with events described in this book have been changed. Any similarity to actual persons is coincidental.

Da Capo Press books are available at special discounts for bulk purchases in the U.S. by corporations, institutions, and other organizations. For more information, please contact the Special Markets Department at the Perseus Books Group, 2300 Chestnut Street, Suite 200, Philadelphia, PA, 19103, or call (800) 810-4145, ext. 5000, or e-mail special.markets@perseusbooks.com.

10 9 8 7 6 5 4

For busy people who love to eat good food and enjoy experiencing cutting-edge cuisine. Here's to your vibrant health and satisfaction—and to spending less time in the kitchen! With many thanks for your support.

Contents

CONTENTS

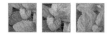

Foreword

By Deborah Madison

Imagine starting the day with a luscious "galactic" smoothie that's filled with dates and papayas, or a chai latte made not from a tea bag or a mix, but from black tea simmered with ginger and spices, the way it's done traditionally. For something more substantial, you might add a southwest scramble—of not eggs, but tofu and herbs and spices—filling, yes, but it's also light. For lunch, you might dip into a warm bowl of soba noodles or make yourself a wrap (add a side of pickled beets here) and, come dinnertime, you may anticipate tucking into a red lentil–infused quinoa kitchari or a warm African sweet potato soup. Need a snack between meals? How about some toasted pepitas, crispy kale (now *this* is good!), or flavored popcorn? Do you have children? There are recipes just for them. Open *The 30-Minute Vegan* and you might well be surprised—and no doubt pleased—by what's inside. A host of appealing recipes can be found between the covers of this book, as well as a lot of good information about food and cooking in general, surprisingly realistic approaches to thirty-minute cooking with real food, and more, from glossaries to Web sites.

The authors, Mark Reinfeld and Jennifer Murray, know that I'm not a vegan and probably you should know that, too. Although butter and cheese find their way into my vegetarian cookbooks and my kitchen, quite a few of my recipes are vegan, too, simply because many dishes I love happen to be so. Traditional, largely plant-based food cultures are full of dishes that today could be called "vegan," and they are the dishes I turned to when I opened Greens restaurant in 1979. Like our vegetarian dishes, they were greeted with enthusiasm, not because they were lacking dairy, but because they tasted good and were familiar to our mostly nonvegetarian customers.

(Who didn't know pesto?) Looking back to that time, it would have been difficult to imagine a vegan menu, or a book like *The 30-Minute Vegan,* which often overlooks traditional flavors in favor of a more carefree blend of elements and ingredients. But I'm open to being open, and I'm delighted to have Mark and Jennifer's book in hand. It's introduced me to some new dishes and although I may never be a full-time vegan—I did grow up on a small dairy farm, after all, and cream is in my veins—I can certainly appreciate recipes that sidestep some ingredients we may well benefit from setting aside at least from time to time, while retaining flavor and appeal.

What I especially appreciate in *The 30-Minute Vegan* is the effort Mark and Jennifer make to woo, albeit gently, the reader away from highly processed convenience foods even if they are vegan, toward foods that are whole, fresh, and minimally processed, which means, one really does need to do some cooking. Although they live and cook in Hawaii, *The 30-Minute Vegan* is not too Hawaii based, which makes it ultimately practical for the home cook who happens to live on the mainland. Add to these virtues the knowledge that you're not going to be spending all day in the kitchen and you have a very useful book, indeed. Because Mark and Jennifer are so committed to helping you put real food on the table in a half hour or less, they provide various tips and tricks, including encouraging readers to hone their knife skills, which is good advice for anyone, but especially for people who haven't spent much time in the kitchen. They also know that if you aren't linear about how you think of cooking and organize yourself, you can accomplish a lot more quickly—more good advice and the kind that's often lacking in thirty-minute cookbooks.

This practical book is also a friendly one. "Use what you have and what you love," the authors advise if you can't find a particular ingredient—a relief for many, I'm sure. And although vegan food may be different from mainstream food, who says that vegans don't want to have some egg(less) nog during the holidays, a chocolate-covered strawberry now and then, or lemon bars? . . . They do, and even if they're not quite like what the rest of us are familiar with, the authors are generous in their offering of vegan approaches to familiar dishes such as corn on the cob, pizzas and pastas, BBQ sauce (for tempeh), polenta, as well as desserts.

For me as a cook, the goal of any cuisine, especially one that omits culturally mainstream ingredients, like animal products, is to come up with food that is delicious and a joy to eat. My favorite comment from customers at Greens was, "Oh, I forgot that there wasn't any meat." You want your eater, even if it's just you, to come away from a meal having forgotten all about those missing ingredients. It's not enough to exclude the shunned ingredient—that's only going partway. The food has to sing, too.

So I especially appreciate that *The 30-Minute Vegan* emphasizes building blocks for flavor, such as herb-infused oils, and even the uses of herbs, so important and so often ignored. That there's an emphasis on food that's fresh, local, seasonal, and organic speaks, not only to our concerns about the environment, but again to the quality of the foods we cook. If you want to cook simply and well, you'll be best off if you cook with the most flavorful ingredients, which, as it happens, tend to be fresh, seasonal, local, and organic. A useful glossary of foods and tools says that cooking know-how is taken seriously here, and it needs to be if you want to be self-reliant and free of processed foods. And I am forever happy that there are no breakdowns of recipes to keep readers obsessive about things one needn't (and no doubt shouldn't) be obsessing about.

Despite the challenges afoot with embracing a vegan lifestyle—not only the decision to be vegan but to fully enjoy eating this way—Mark and Jennifer offer a calm sense of purpose, unquestionable joy, and warm encouragement to those who want to cook and eat this way—especially those who find time in short supply.

Deborah Madison
author of Vegetarian Cooking for Everyone

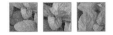

Preface

One of the most pressing issues of our time is how to deal with our busyness. No matter where we go these days, people feel busier than ever. It affects our health, our happiness, our relationships, and virtually every part of our lives. Too often it feels like a stretch to even spend time with the people we love—not to mention learning a new way of eating, even if we do crave more health and vitality.

We created *30-Minute Vegan* out of a sincere desire to address this issue for anyone willing to devote just a little bit of their precious time. This book is a bounty of quick and easy, delectable vegan cuisine for busy people. We are a husband and wife team living in Hawaii. We enjoy spending time in the kitchen together and we never tire of bossing each other around. We aspire to impart some of our culinary enthusiasm to you.

We've selected recipes that illustrate the diversity yet simplicity and ease of vegan food preparation. Here you will find healthful recipes for every occasion—from romantic dinners for two to slumber parties for your children. You'll find lots of suggestions for recipe modifications; you can be adventurous and still be time savvy. If you're a novice in the kitchen, playing with these recipes will help you become more comfortable with cooking. Seasoned chefs can delight in some of our time-saving techniques while discovering new tastes by being inventive with the variations.

Superfoods for Health

One of our guiding principles is that food is best when enjoyed in its whole, natural state. This goes for both flavor and nutritional quality. **Superfoods** are those foods that are packed with nutrients and have been shown to have outstanding health benefits. Many of these are ancient foods that have been revered for thousands of years for their healing qualities. They are high in disease-fighting antioxidants, which are known to protect cells from damage, even slowing down the aging process in many instances. We highlight these wonder foods throughout the book and show how they represent the wave of the future in terms of reclaiming our health.

Organic food is grown without the use of chemical fertilizers and pesticides, many of which have not been fully tested for their effects on humans. Although people continue to debate whether these chemicals are harmful, we know they are not necessary, so we don't take the risk. We highly recommend using organic ingredients whenever possible in our recipes.

Raw or living foods are nutrient-rich foods that have not been heated above 116°F. Live food cuisine is a growing trend in the culinary world. People who eat raw foods report feeling increased energy, weight loss, healing, and a host of other benefits. We indicate the raw food recipes in the book with a ♥.

The importance of eating **locally grown foods** whenever possible cannot be overemphasized. *Locavore* was even recently selected as "new word of the year." It refers to one who eats only local foods. Eating local foods ensures freshness and saves those resources involved in shipping across long distances.

Growing foods in your own garden or participating in community-supported agriculture programs (CSAs) is the best option if you have the opportunity. It's very rewarding to see something grow from seed to plant. Farmers' markets are the next best choice. Make friends with the people growing your food! Many of the recipes in this book can be adapted to include whatever fresh ingredients you have on hand.

Our general approach in the kitchen emphasizes minimizing the use of processed and packaged foods. Not only is this much better for your health, the reduction in packaging is good for the planet as well. In our recipes, we often list homemade alternatives to packaged products, such as to canned beans, commercially made vegan mayonnaise, or sour cream. For your comfort and pleasure, we do include some of our favorite processed "transition foods," such as vegan cream cheese and vegan butter for those just beginning to include more plant-based foods or for special occasions.

Going Green with Vegan Cuisine

A **vegetarian** diet is one that does not include meat, fish, or poultry. **Vegan** food contains no animal products or by-products. It's vegetarian without the dairy or eggs. For this reason, vegan cuisine is often referred to as "plant-based." The reasons people choose to enjoy vegan foods are many. First and foremost, vegan foods taste incredible, as you will discover when you sample the recipes in this book. People also turn to vegan foods for weight loss and disease prevention. Numerous studies show that many illnesses, such as diabetes, heart disease, certain forms of cancer, and obesity can be prevented and reversed with appropriate changes in diet and lifestyle.

A plant-based diet also helps protect the environment. Now with more attention than ever on global warming and greenhouse gases, people are realizing that making changes to our diet is the most effective impact we can have on our planet. The environmental footprint of a vegan diet is a fraction of that of a meat-based diet. A recent United Nations report, *Livestock's Long Shadow*, shows that 18 percent of all greenhouse gas emissions come from the livestock industry, more than the entire world's transportation industry combined!

Vegan foods represent the best utilization of the earth's limited resources. It takes 16 pounds of grain and 2,500 gallons of water to produce a single pound of beef. It's astonishing that the beef industry continues to flourish when we see so much in the news about food and water shortages and people going to bed hungry. For more information on veganism and organic foods, please see appendix A.

About VeganFusion.com

Vegan Fusion World Cuisine is a style of food preparation that draws upon culinary traditions from around the globe. In our books and classes, we share tips and tricks based on years of experience at our restaurants and feedback from countless customers.

Visit our Web site, VeganFusion.com, to learn about the vegan lifestyle, sign up for our free newsletter, and find out more about our books: *Vegan Fusion World Cuisine* (the winner of nine national awards, including a Gourmand Award for Best Vegetarian Cookbook in the USA, Best New Cookbook by PETA, and Cookbook of the Year by VegNews) and *The Complete Idiot's Guide to Eating Raw*.

How to Use This Book

The recipes in each chapter are more or less listed from "lighter" to "heavier." Virtually all of the recipes can be completed in less than thirty minutes, including preparation and cooking time. Several recipes do have cooking or baking times that exceed this time frame, but the labor time is under thirty minutes in every case. You'll find that we've also included many exciting variations to the recipes, some of which may also take longer than thirty minutes. These are clearly noted. The clock starts ticking once the ingredients have been gathered and are ready for use. The time doesn't include searching through the cabinets for tools or ingredients.

Read through the recipe carefully, perhaps even twice. Make sure you have everything you need and gather it before you begin. Also remember that with practice, everything becomes easier. The more you make a recipe, the faster you will become.

Use these recipes as a starting point for creating your own versions and specialties based on your preferences and whatever ingredients you have on hand. We strongly encourage creative expression in the kitchen; don't just try to stick to the recipe. Never let one or two missing ingredients stop you from making a recipe. There is always something you can substitute—be creative!

Create the Space

We encourage you to create an inspiring ambience when you prepare your meals. Listening to your favorite music and bringing flowers or other objects of beauty into the kitchen will help spark your culinary creativity. We sincerely hope that *30-Minute Vegan* motivates you to prepare more of your own vegan food and to share a meal with loved ones. Celebrate the flavors and the ease of these recipes. Have fun and enjoy the process!

To Life!
Mark and Jennifer

the
30 Minute
Vegan

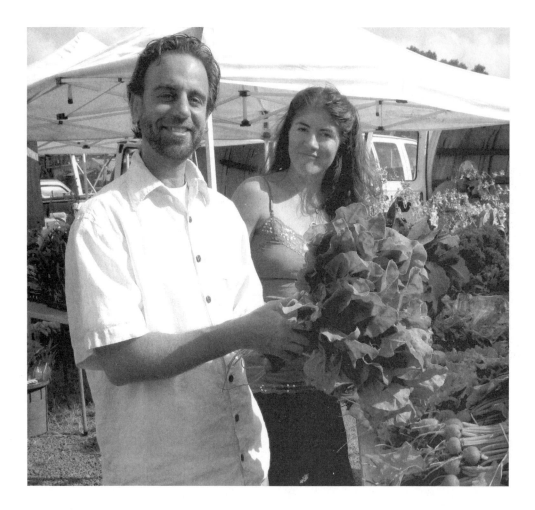

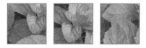

CHAPTER I

Getting Started

Before you dive into the recipes, let's go over some essentials. This chapter highlights our favorite ingredients to help you set up a rocking vegan pantry. We also go over some of the kitchen gear that will help you along your way. Finally, we have a list of tips and tricks for kitchen efficiency and tastiness. Consult this list frequently!

As you go through the recipes, you will be learning many of the basic techniques involved in natural food preparation. These techniques are detailed in chapter 2.

Shopping

Try shopping on your least busy day and make an adventure of it. If you become familiar with your local farmers' market and health food store, you'll find shopping is an enjoyable adventure. Spend lots of time in the produce aisle and sample different fruits and vegetables as they become available seasonally. Educate yourself by reading labels. If you are having trouble pronouncing ingredients, it could be that artificial ones lurk within the package.

When shopping for produce, look for vibrant colors with a bit of firmness. When shopping for nuts, seeds, grains, and beans, purchase only what you're going to consume within a few weeks. Nuts and seeds should have a crunch to them.

We always recommend enjoying foods as soon after preparing them as possible. Some dishes actually do taste better the next day, once the flavors have had a chance to deepen. The recipes in this book generally keep for at least two or three days if stored properly, and certain items such as dressings keep for up to a week or longer.

The Vegan Pantry . . . Ingredients Galore!

So many awesome flavors await you! You don't need to go out and purchase all of these ingredients at once. Build your pantry over time. The more variety of foods you have access to, the more motivated you will be to try new dishes. All of these ingredients are available at health food stores. Many large supermarkets now have a "natural food" section (makes you wonder what kind of food is in the rest of the store) or integrate natural foods throughout the store. You can also check out appendix B for Web sites where you can place special orders online.

Remember to go for local and organic ingredients whenever possible. Visit ethnic markets to experience the diversity of culinary traditions. See the glossary for more information on many of these ingredients.

Consider stocking up on some of these essentials:

Fruits: Fresh fruits are the ideal snack. You will appreciate having many types on hand, including lemons and limes, which are excellent on salads and with drinking water. Dried fruits are also fabulous for quick snacks and natural sweeteners. Sample some of the many dates available, such as Medjool, Deglet Noor, or Barhi. We like to keep dates soaking in water in the refrigerator, for use in smoothies and desserts. We also love figs (black mission, Turkish, Calimyrna), raisins, apricots, and cranberries. Store dry fruits in an airtight glass container in a cool, dry place, or in the refrigerator.

You may also wish to have some store-bought organic lemon or lime juice on hand, especially when making larger batches of dishes that call for the juice. The Santa Cruz Organic juice company puts out a good product.

Vegetables: Staples include mixed salad greens, kale, carrots, onion, celery, potatoes, and garlic. A steamed veggie medley is just moments away with such veggies as broccoli, cauliflower, and zucchini. You may wish to consider stocking some frozen vegetables, such as peas, carrots, corn, and spinach, for when you are really in a crunch for time. Dried chiles are an amazing addition for Mexican, Indian, and Southwestern dishes. Try different varieties, such as Serrano, chipotle, ancho, and guajillo.

Herbs: You'll be surprised when you find out how easy it is to have your own herb garden right in your kitchen. Most herbs grow well in pots and have a long history, rich with folklore and medicinal use. Sample herbs one at a time to learn their characteristics. Try different combinations to discover flavors you like. It's a trial-and-error exploration, so have fun with it. Consider experimenting with fresh culinary herbs such as basil, dill, oregano, thyme, rosemary, lemongrass, chives, mints, cilantro (coriander), marjoram, sage, chervil, turmeric, kaffir lime leaves, bay leaves, tarragon (French and Mexican varieties), Thai basil, and flat-leaf Italian parsley.

If a recipe calls for fresh herbs and all you have is dried, you can substitute. Use 1 teaspoon of dried herb for every 1 tablespoon of fresh herb called for in the recipe.

Spices: Getting to know your different spices and spice combinations is an ongoing adventure. Expertise comes with practice over time as you build upon your knowledge. Consider stocking your pantry with these popular dried culinary spices: cumin, chile powder (see Note), cinnamon, cloves, curry powder, turmeric, ginger, coriander (dried cilantro), cardamom, fenugreek, mustard seeds, fennel seeds, nutmeg, black pepper, saffron, cayenne, paprika, allspice, and aniseed.

Note: For recipes that call for chile powder: you can use the available chile powder blends, which contain ground chile as well as cumin, garlic, and other spices. If so, make sure you are using a salt-free variety. You can also use pure ground chile powder (molido), which is made only with ground chiles. Please keep in mind that this pure ground chile is spicier than the blends.

Nuts and Seeds: Purchase the raw varieties and store them in airtight glass jars in a cool, dark place, even the refrigerator or freezer if you have the space. Some of our favorite nuts include almonds, walnuts, pecans, macadamia nuts, cashews, hazelnuts (filberts), pine nuts, pistachios, walnuts, and almonds. For seeds, try sunflower, pumpkin, sesame (the unhulled variety), flax, and hemp. We also like to have ground flaxseeds on hand for juices and for several recipes in this book. Place flaxseeds in a blender or spice grinder and grind to a fine meal. Store the flax meal in an airtight glass container in the refrigerator for up to a week.

Grains and Legumes: Quite a few grains can be cooked and enjoyed within thirty minutes. These include quinoa, oats, buckwheat, amaranth, millet, and white basmati rice. Other important grains to include are short- and long-grain brown rice, brown basmati rice, black rice, and barley. Although these grains take longer than thirty minutes to cook, the amount of time required to prepare them is actually less than five minutes. Please see the grain cooking chart in chapter 2 for more information on cooking grains.

Regarding legumes, red lentils can cook in less than thirty minutes. Other favorites that take longer than thirty minutes include black beans, pinto beans, kidney beans, black-eyed peas, navy beans, lentils (green, yellow, and French), and mung beans. Prepare beans in advance or have cans on hand for when you are pressed for time. Refer to the legume cooking chart in chapter 2 for information on cooking legumes.

Salts: We recommend sea salt over iodized table salt, which is highly refined and contains anticaking agents. Celtic sea salt is a widely acclaimed unprocessed whole salt from France. Himalayan crystal salt is another popular choice. For brevity, in our recipes, we list salt as "sea salt" to distinguish it from table salt. Most of the recipes that call for salt suggest adding it to taste.

Sweeteners: Refined white sugar is implicated in many illnesses. The good news is that there are many natural sweet tastes to choose from. Try these less-refined natural sweeteners: agave nectar or syrup, stevia leaf, maple syrup, Sucanat (stands for sugar cane natural), turbinado sugar, molasses, barley malt syrup, brown rice syrup, and yakon syrup. See the glossary for more explanation of these natural sweeteners.

Sea vegetables or seaweeds: These make an important addition to the vegan pantry. In addition to providing vital minerals and nutrients, they also impart a seafood flavor to dishes. Try dulse, arame, hijiki, kombu, wakame, nori sheets, and kelp. Store sea veggies in an airtight container in a cool, dark place. Also, a versatile new product is on the market: kelp noodles from Sea Tangle Noodle Company, which is a refrigerated item.

Oils: For maximum freshness, to minimize oxidation and prevent the oil from becoming rancid, be sure your oils are cold pressed and stored in dark jars.

Choose cold-pressed, extra-virgin olive oil. It's from the first pressing and is rich in flavor and nutrients. Other oils to consider include sesame (toasted and light), coconut, sunflower, and safflower.

For salads, we like flaxseed oil and hemp oil. These oils have a nutty flavor and are plant-based sources of essential fatty acids. They require refrigeration and are not meant to be heated. You can also try borage and pumpkin seed oils.

Vinegars: Most vinegar lasts about two years in a cool, dark place. Once opened, use within six months to a year, for best flavor. Our favorite vinegar is raw unfiltered apple cider vinegar, which also has a rich folklore for treating many ailments. Other vinegars to sample include balsamic, red wine, unfiltered brown rice vinegar, umeboshi plum vinegar, and more exotic vinegars such as raspberry or champagne. See page 284 to discover how to create your own herbal vinegars.

Water: We cannot overstate the importance of using pure, clean water. We recommend using filtered water for all of our recipes. High-quality tap water can be used if filtered water is unavailable. In the interest of reducing plastics and waste, consider investing in a water filter available through Web sites in the "Eco-Friendly Products & Services" section of appendix B. Contemplate this: Our body is comprised of 70 to 80 percent water. We are what we drink!

Breads and Flours: For breads, check out Nature's Path's Manna Bread, which is made from sprouted grains and baked at low temperatures. We also like sprouted whole-grain breads and tortillas. As for flours, spelt and buckwheat are our favorites. Spelt is an ancient variety of wheat. However, please note that it is not gluten-free and may not be tolerated by those allergic to wheat. Buckwheat is both wheat- and gluten-free.

Pastas and Noodles: Brown rice pasta is our favorite. Tinkyada puts out a superior product. Experiment with different shapes and sizes. Also check out Japanese noodles such as soba, which is made from buckwheat, and udon, made from wheat. Read noodle ingredients carefully to be sure the product does not contain lactose.

Tofu and Tempeh: Tofu is processed soybean curd and has its origins in ancient China. It comes in several forms, including extra-firm, firm, soft, and silken. Our recipes indicate which type is called for. Recently, you can even find sprouted tofu. The sprouting makes the tofu easier to digest while the flavor is much the same.

Tempeh is originally from Indonesia. It consists of soybeans fermented in a rice culture, then cooked. Many different varieties are created by mixing the soybean with grains, such as millet, wheat, or rice, and with sea vegetables and seasonings. Tempeh has a heavier, courser texture than tofu. It usually has a mild, slightly fermented flavor. Its color is usually tan with a few dark gray spots. Tempeh needs to be thoroughly cooked by either steaming, sautéing, roasting, or grilling. To store, tempeh may be frozen or refrigerated.

Condiments and Special Treats

Condiments are a simple way to enhance the flavor of dishes. We provide recipes for many of our favorites in chapter 13. Check out your local health food stores or comprehensive Web sites, such as www.sunfood.com or www.goldmine.com, for a wealth of vegan condiments.

Here are some more staples to include:

Nut and seed butters: Try almond, cashew, and macadamia. They are available in many health food stores. We also love tahini, a creamy butter made from ground sesame seeds, which is a staple in Middle Eastern cuisine. A few companies dedicated to raw foods will grind their nuts and seeds slowly over the course of a few days to keep the temperature from becoming too high. Coconut butter is another favorite for smoothies and desserts.

Red Star's Nutritional Yeast: One of our favorite condiments, it's a vegan source of protein and vitamin B_{12} that adds a cheeselike and nutty flavor to dishes. Store nutritional yeast in a cool, dark place in an airtight jar, and use it within a few months.

Mirin: A sweet rice wine that imparts a depth and sweet flavor to dishes. It is often used as that special "secret ingredient," combining well with the saltiness of soy sauce. When you don't have mirin, you can substitute a fifty-fifty combination of apple juice and rice wine vinegar, sherry, or even brown rice vinegar to achieve a similar effect.

Miso paste: A staple in Japanese cuisine that's made from cultured soybeans, rice, or barley. The culturing process creates enzymes and many beneficial nutrients such as B-vitamins and essential amino acids. Be sure to purchase the unpasteurized variety. Miso varies in color from light varieties, such as mellow, shiro, or garbanzo bean miso to the darker ones, such as brown rice, hatcho, red, or barley miso. The lighter varieties are usually fermented for a shorter period and are more delicately flavored and sometimes sweet. The darker varieties are heavier and saltier.

Soy sauces: Nama Shoyu is an unpasteurized soy sauce (*nama* means "raw" in Japanese) made from cultured soybeans and wheat. We list Nama Shoyu as the soy sauce in our raw recipes. For the cooked recipes, we like to use tamari, a wheat-free soy sauce. Feel free to replace the soy sauce listed in the recipes with Shoyu, tamari, or a soy sauce of your choosing.

Nondairy milks: Soy, rice, almond, and hemp milk are healthful alternatives to cow's milk. There are many varieties on the market, so try a few to find your favorite. See chapter 3 for homemade seed and nut milks.

Baking and dessert ingredients: To explore the world of desserts, stock up on baking soda, baking powder, grain-sweetened dairy-free chocolate and carob chips, dairy-free cocoa powder, vanilla extract (preferably alcohol-free), and flavorings such as mint, raspberry, orange, almond, coffee, banana, hazelnut, and more. Also consider a few specialty items such as tapioca flour (or Egg Replacer by Ener-G Foods), shredded coconut, rosewater and other food grade hydrosols.

Superfood condiments: Culinary superfood supplements that we add to smoothies and live desserts include raw cacao powder and nibs, spirulina, maca powder, and raw carob powder. Fresh vanilla beans add gourmet flair to smoothies and desserts. Try the Tahitian and Mexican varieties.

Japanese condiments: Pickled ginger, wasabi powder, and umeboshi plum paste are available at most health food stores and Asian foods markets. Use pickled ginger and its brine to add an extra exotic flare to dishes. Wasabi, the green spicy mustard paste you get with sushi, can be used to add a deep spicy twist. Umeboshi plum paste is very tangy and salty; it takes a little getting used to. It is revered in macrobiotic food preparation for its health promoting properties.

Transition condiments: These we don't recommend consuming on a regular basis. Use in moderation to satisfy a craving for their less healthy dairy alternatives. Follow Your Heart is a company that makes Vegenaise, an outstanding vegan mayo. They also have a superior vegan mozzarella and cream cheese. Earth Balance tops the list for dairy-free butter replacers. Teese makes an awesome vegan mozzarella. You can also try Vegan Gourmet brand cheeses, which include Cheddar and Monterey Jack flavors. Tofutti's Better than Cream Cheese is a good choice if you are totally craving cream cheese. Tofutti also makes a vegan sour cream. For vegan yogurt, try the Silk brand, which has many flavors, or Nancy's, which makes a nice sugar-free variety.

Other special foods to stock up on include granola, pasta sauce, tomato paste, curry paste (check out Thai Kitchen's product), coconut milk (beware of cream of coconut, which may contain dairy products), and cans of your favorite beans. Of course, there are old favorite condiments such as ketchup and mustard. *30-Minute Vegan* chefs will also find it helpful to have a salad dressing on hand—either homemade or a store-bought variety.

Kitchen Gear

Many gadgets and utensils make cooking fun—and easy. It's exciting and sparks creativity to have a wide selection of tools to work with. As with the vegan pantry, build your kitchen gear over time as your means allow.

Here are some essentials to begin with:

Knives: A good knife is the single most important tool in the kitchen. Having a reliable sharp blade to work with makes the difference between an enjoyable experience and a highly unpleasant one. It is less likely for an injury to occur when using a sharp blade. Follow the manufacturer's guidelines when it comes to sharpening and storing knives.

Start with an 8-inch chef knife. Other knives to include are a paring knife, for garnishes and peeling, and a serrated knife, which is handy for slicing bread and tomatoes. For stainless-steel knives, we like Henckels, Wusthof, and Victorinox. You may wish to consider investing in ceramic knives. They're sharper than most steel knives, and they can last for years without sharpening. Ceramic knife blades are lightweight, easy to clean, leave no metallic taste or smell, and are stain- and rust-proof. Check out the Kyocera and Shenzhen brands.

Blender: We recommend investing in a good blender. You will thank yourself every time you whip up a smoothie or creamy pudding. They are also ideal for dressings, creamy soups, sauces, frostings, and spreads. Hamilton Beach makes a decent household brand. Vita-Mix and Blendtec's Total Blender are top-of-the-line choices.

Toaster oven: This is a must-have for the *30-Minute Vegan* kitchen. It takes less time to heat up, uses less energy, and cooks food faster than a regular oven. Many quick and easy dishes can be prepared on the baking tray.

Food processor: This is the tool to use for pâtés and spreads, and for grating large quantities of carrots, beets, cabbage, and other veggies. Cuisinart is a popular brand. There are even mini food processors, which come in handy for mincing garlic, chopping small amounts of nuts, or making small portions of spreads so you don't need to get the big one dirty.

Juicer: Some recommended brands include Green Star, which sells possibly the best juicer in terms of minimal loss of nutrition. It extracts the juice of virtually anything, even wheatgrass, without needing to change parts. It can also process nuts, seeds, and grains. The Champion Juicer is another classic and it can be used to make nut butters and all-fruit ice creams. The Breville brand is another popular and highly rated juicer.

Here is a checklist of other gear, from aprons to zesters, to consider as you accessorize your kitchen:

Apron (bring your fashion sense to the kitchen)

Baking sheets and casserole dishes—avoid aluminum; we like stoneware

Bamboo sushi mat, for nori rolls

Basting brush

Cast-iron or stainless-steel pots and pans of various sizes (no aluminum or Teflon). You can start with a 3-quart pot, a 5-quart pot, and a medium-size sauté pan and build from there. Also, most stores offer a starter pack with several pots and pans, which is a great way to begin.

Cheesecloth or fine-mesh bags, for straining nut milks and other liquids

Citrus juicer—we use a handheld one that fits onto a small glass jar

Colander

Cutting board—we like bamboo or wood

Dehydrator, for live food preparation (see glossary)

Garlic press—it's worth getting a high-quality one

Ginger grater

Glass containers with airtight lids, for refrigerated and other food storage

Grater—commonly referred to as a cheese grater; can be used for grating many vegetables as well as zesting citrus in a pinch

Griddle/grill—a useful item that straddles two burners and has a griddle on one side (you can make four pancakes at once!) and grooves on the other side (for grilling)

Hand blender, for making creamy soups without using a full-size blender.

Hand towels

Kitchen scissors, for harvesting fresh herbs and opening packaging

Mandoline—enables you to slice, julienne, and waffle-cut your favorite vegetables. The blade is razor sharp, so pay attention when slicing.

Measuring cups and spoons

Mixing bowls—use nonreactive metal or glass, not plastic

Oven mitts and pot holders

Salad spinner

Scoops of various sizes, including a small melon scoop

Slow cooker, such as Crock-Pot

Spatulas—wood and firm plastic ones

Spice grinder (a.k.a. coffee grinder) and/or a mortar and pestle, for grinding spices and seeds

Spiralizers—the Saladacco or Spiral Slicer spiralizer turns zucchini, yams, carrots, and any other firm vegetable into angel hair "pasta," wide flat ribbons, or thin slices

Steamer basket—use one of bamboo or stainless steel

Strainers—you can get very cheap fine-mesh ones at most drugstores and they come in very handy. Usually they have plastic handles with wire mesh and come in a set of two or three. Or look for stainless-steel strainers, which are sturdier and rustproof.

Vegetable peeler

Whisks

Zester—one of our favorite tools is the Microplane fine grater that grates citrus peels and spices into ultrafine zests

The Pen Is as Mighty as the Fork

Keeping a food journal is an effective way to chart your progress in the kitchen. Use it to record your recipe creation process, comments on ingredients, herb and spice combinations, farmer or farmers' market and health food store contact information, and any other kitchen revelations. If your goal is to lose weight, a recent study revealed that the simple act of writing down foods eaten during the day can double the amount of pounds you lose. You can also track your food intake on Web sites such as www.myfooddiary.com or www.nutritiondata.com, which offer nutritional data and sample meal plans.

A Word about the Recipes

Our recipes are selected with the idea of transitioning in mind. This means to hold a vision of where you would like to be with your diet and take steps to get there. We offer vegan recipes that range from heavier comfort foods (we even have a whole chapter devoted to this) to "lighter" raw foods. We do include recipes with soy cheese or vegan mayonnaise as transition foods for those accustomed to the flavor and texture of animal-based dishes. We encourage you to gravitate toward lighter foods and your body will thank you.

Sidebars

Throughout the pages you will see the following sidebars:

If You Have More Time: these recipes and variations of recipes take longer than thirty minutes. If you have time to explore them, you will be well rewarded.

Quicker and Easier: while the whole book may be considered quick and easy, these recipes are even quicker and easier to prepare.

Superfoods for Health: these sidebars highlight some of our favorite super-foods and describe how they contribute to optimal health.

Tips and Tricks: learn the secrets of the pros that make your life in the kitchen easier and more fun.

10 Keys to Success in the Kitchen: Guidelines for Quickness & Accuracy

Remember that food is an art . . . these tips will help you have great success in the kitchen and will enable you to enjoy yourself. If you're having a good time, everyone will enjoy the results no matter what.

1. Read each recipe thoroughly. Look up words and ingredients you are unfamiliar with in our glossary or a dictionary. Understand the process involved. Understand when multitasking is necessary rather than waiting for each step to be complete before moving on to the next step.

2. Before beginning any preparation, create a clean work area. Gather the ingredients in the recipe before you start. This ensures that you have everything you need, that you will know what you will be using as a substitute (if necessary), and eliminates time spent searching through cabinets. Gather your measuring spoons and cups, tools, and appliances. Preparing food in a clean and organized space is always easier.

3. Having the proper tools is essential to being able to whip food up quickly. It may increase your cooking time if you don't have tools such as a garlic press, zester, citrus juicer, or blender. Work up to a fully stocked kitchen.

4. Although the recipes are designed to taste their best by your following the exact measurements, eventually you will learn to discover acceptable approximations. At some point you will be able to look at two different cloves of garlic and know that one is about one teaspoon, and the other is about one tablespoon. In cases like these, don't worry too much about measuring everything with ultimate precision. With baking, however, measurements need to be precise, since leavening is involved.

5. Some herbs, such as parsley, cilantro, or fennel, don't need to be plucked from the thin part of their stems before mincing or chopping. Just keep them bundled together and chop into the whole bunch at once. The thin parts of the stems generally have the same flavor and, once minced, basically taste the same.

6. Cut stacks of veggies rather than each individual piece. Don't separate celery stalks when you can cut into the whole bunch at once. The same goes for heads of lettuce and cabbage. Stack tomato, potato, or onion slices and cut them simultaneously.

7. The easiest way to sift flour is with a fine-mesh strainer. For accuracy, always sift baking soda, baking powder, cocoa powder, and any spices that have lumps.

8. You don't need to peel carrots, cucumbers, potatoes, zucchini, or beets unless specified; just wash them well. This is not only quicker but also helps preserve the nutritional content of the food.

9. Most blenders have cup and fluid ounce measurements right on the pitcher; no need to dirty more measuring cups.

10. One of the most important tips to help cut down on preparation time is to set aside an hour or so on one of your least busy days for advance prepping. Having prepped ingredients on hand makes it easier to create meals on the go. Here you can cut vegetables and store them in a glass container in the fridge. You can also cook a squash, grain, or pot of beans. You can then use these foods in recipes over the next few days. Consider preparing a pot of rice in the morning and using it for the evening meal.

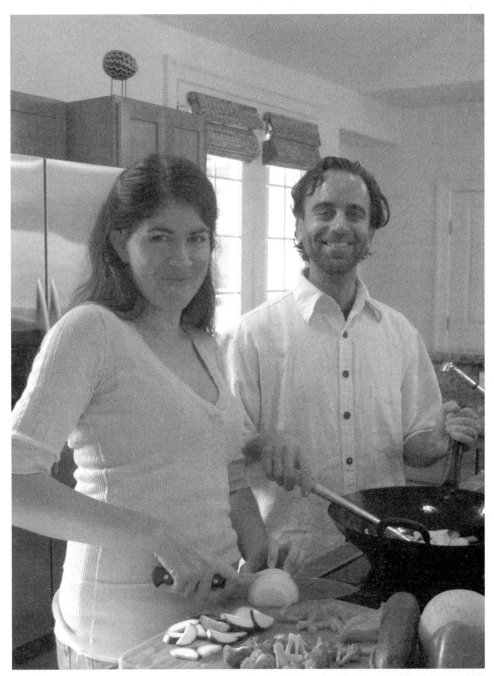

(Photo by Dawn Reinfeld)

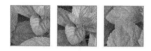

CHAPTER 2

Preparation Basics

This chapter is our Vegan Prep 101. These techniques, tips, and tricks are referred to throughout *The 30-Minute Vegan* and are included here to give you a basic understanding of everything you need to know to create world-class vegan cuisine. The three most important things to remember are practice, practice, and practice. Once you become more adept in the kitchen, you'll find it's a snap to create healthy, delicious dishes in under thirty minutes. If you are patient and persistent, you will succeed.

Knife Work

Working with a knife is one of the most basic skills to cultivate in the kitchen. Expertise comes with practice. To help you along the way, you can check out the Food Network's educational online video demonstrations of various knife techniques, at www.foodnetwork.com/food/ck_dm_knife_skills.

Here is a brief description of the most common cuts:

Mince: cut into tiny pieces, the finest cut that can be cut by hand.
Dice: slightly larger than minced, usually ¼-inch uniform pieces.
Chop: larger than diced, can be various sizes. Typically ½ inch in diameter and larger.

Slice: many types are possible—thin or thick, half-moon shaped, rings, or diagonal.

Cube: chopped into uniform squares; can be various sizes.

Julienne: long and thin strips, approximately ⅛-inch wide.

Chiffonade: long, thinly cut strips of herbs or leafy veggies, achieved by rolling them up and then slicing.

Shred: cut into very thin strips, either by hand or by using a grater or food processor.

In your spare time, you can also practice turning fruits and vegetables into beautiful garnishes—an art form in itself. Experiment with different colors and sizes as you decorate your plates before serving. Carrots can be cut into stars; radishes and beets into roses; and many other intriguing forms await your knife as you become more experienced. Visit www.recipetips.com and do a keyword search for "garnishing" to learn several unique techniques.

Steaming

Steaming involves using a steamer basket made of either bamboo or stainless steel. Vegetables are placed in the basket; the basket is placed in a pot with 1 to 2 inches of water; and the pot is covered with a lid. As the water boils, the vegetables are cooked in the steam that is generated by the boiling water. Lightly steaming preserves as much of the foods' nutritional value as possible. A small steamer basket fits well in a 3-quart pot and can provide countless quick and easy steamed veggie medleys.

If several vegetables are used, place the firmer vegetables that take longer to cook, such as yams, carrots, and cauliflower, in the steamer first and steam for a few minutes. (Also place on the lowest level of the steamer any vegetables whose juices may color or add an unpleasant taste to other vegetables they'd sit atop, such as beets or Brussels sprouts.) Add other vegetables such as broccoli, green beans, red bell peppers, mushrooms, purple cabbage, zucchini, or snow peas, and cook until just tender. Check periodically to make sure you don't run out of water. Experiment with different timings to discover how long it takes to cook them to perfection.

With regard to measurements: Generally, 1 cup of raw vegetables will yield 1 cup of cooked vegetables, if not overcooked. For the more tender leafy greens, such as spinach or Swiss chard, 1 cup of raw veggies will yield approximately ½ cup or less steamed.

Blanching

Sometimes we like to precook hardier veggies such as broccoli or cauliflower before using them in a sauté or as crudités and in salads. This involves dipping the veggies in boiling water for several seconds to a few minutes, and then placing them immediately into ice water. This helps stop the cooking process and imparts a vibrant fresh color to vegetables.

Sometimes, we **blanch almonds** to remove their skins. Timing is important, especially for live food dishes. Drop the soaked almonds in boiling water, remove after 10 seconds, drain, and rinse well under cold water before removing the skins. The skins will easily pop off after blanching. The longer the almonds are left in the water, the less "live" they will be.

Sautéing

Sautéing involves cooking in a pan at a high temperature, usually with oil added. It is recommended to heat the pan before adding the oil. You can use a sauté pan or try using a wok. This is the technique used in the famous stir-fry—with all its variations. If you do use a wok, remember the sides of the wok are cooler than the bottom. As you add new veggies to your stir-fry, move the cooked ones to the side to allow the newer ones to cook on the hotter surface.

In your sautéing, avoid at all costs using any of the hydrogenated oils. These oils are damaging to heart health. There are so many wonderful nonhydrogenated oils out there—this book suggests many of them. Reap their benefits for your health and taste buds! Our favorite oils for sautéing include coconut, olive, sesame, and safflower. Be sure to avoid heating any oil until it smokes. This "smoke point" indicates that the oil has been denatured and is detrimental to health.

Steam Sautéing

Steam sautéing may be used by those wishing to eliminate the use of heated oils in their food. Water or stock is used instead of oil in the initial cooking stages for dishes that are sautéed. Everything else with the recipe, including timings and measurements, is the same as if you were using oil. Place a small amount of water or stock in a heated pan, add vegetables, and follow the recipes as you would if using oil. Add small amounts of water at a time if necessary, to prevent sticking. Lemon juice may also be mixed with the water for added flavor.

Roasting Vegetables

You will be amazed at how this simple technique brings out a deep, rich flavor to vegetables that enhances any dish. The length of time to roast will depend on the type and size of the vegetables. Softer vegetables, such as corn or zucchini, will take close to ten minutes, whereas some of the root vegetables, if cut into large pieces, will take longer than thirty. To roast veggies, follow these simple steps.

1. Preheat the oven to 400°F.
2. The veggies can be marinated (see page 21), mixed with olive oil and spices or herbs, or simply cooked in a bit of water and their own juices.
3. Place the vegetables in a casserole dish or on a baking sheet, and place in the oven.
4. Stir occasionally to make sure the vegetables are cooking evenly. There is no hard-and-fast rule for the length of time to roast. Roast until just tender and a knife can pass easily through the center of the veggies.

Some of our favorite vegetables to roast include root vegetables, such as beet, potato, carrot, yam, parsnip, Jerusalem artichoke, and radish. Zucchini, corn, garlic, and bell peppers are also popular choices that roast faster than the root veggies. You can also experiment with roasting at a lower temperature for longer periods of time to add even more depth of flavor to your dish. As far as marinades, newbies can start simply with olive oil, salt, and pepper, and experiment from there.

For **roasted garlic**, you can peel the garlic and roast the cloves as mentioned above, or you can roast them while they are still in their skins and remove the skins afterward. Another method, which usually takes longer than thirty minutes, involves slicing the top ½-inch portion off the stem of a bulb of garlic and placing it in a very small baking dish, sliced side up, topped with olive oil, a pinch of salt and fresh ground pepper, and 1 teaspoon of minced fresh herbs, baking until a knife can easily pass through the garlic, approximately 35 minutes. Squeeze the garlic out of the bulb and use it as a spread for toast or flax crackers, or to enhance the flavor of other spreads, stir-fries, and casseroles.

For **roasted bell peppers**, a quick method is to place them over the flame on a gas stove. Using tongs, flip periodically to ensure even cooking. Cook until char marks appear on the skin. For those without a gas stove, you can roast peppers in the oven at 400°F. This method also may take longer than 30 minutes. Rinse the peppers and place them on a well-oiled baking sheet. Place them in the oven, skin side up, and cook until the skin is charred and bubbly, approximately 35 minutes. Alternatively, you can roast the peppers on the high broil setting. Make five or six 1-inch slices along the top and bottom of the peppers to flatten them out, place on a well-oiled baking tray, and broil for 10 to 15 minutes, or until the skins are charred black. Once peppers are cooked according to your preferred method, place them in a brown paper bag or a covered bowl for 10 minutes. Peel off the skin and remove the seeds.

Marinating

Marinade ingredients significantly determine the flavors of a dish. The main rule of thumb is the longer an ingredient sits in the marinade, the more of its flavors it will acquire. Simply placing tofu or a Portobello mushroom in different marinades creates dramatically different taste sensations. If possible, allow more time for marinating than the recipe calls for. Up to an hour or more will yield a more flavorful dish.

There is vast room for creative experimentation when it comes to marinades. Some of our favorite marinade ingredients include: soy sauce, toasted sesame oil, coconut or olive oil, brown rice vinegar, mirin, mustard, minced garlic or ginger, lemon or lime juices, maple syrup, balsamic vinegar, and a variety of spices and herbs. You can also add sliced or chopped yellow or green onions.

Check out our suggested marinades and be creative with the variations! Experiment with Balsamic Marinade (page 303), Lemon-Herb Marinade (page 121), Live Shoyu Marinade (page 219), and Tahini Marinade (page 224). You can also use sauces, such as BBQ Sauce (page 000) and Spicy Peanut Sauce (page 123), as marinades.

Cooking Grains

Grains are the staple food for many of the world's cultures. A source of fiber, minerals, and B vitamins, these complex carbohydrate foods provide energy to keep us going. Whole grains contain oil that can become rancid and attract insects if not stored correctly. To store grains, keep them in a tightly sealed container in a cool, dry location. They can be stored in a refrigerator for up to three months and in a freezer for up to six months. Cooked grains may be kept in the refrigerator for up to three days.

Follow these three easy steps to cook grains:

1. Rinse the grain thoroughly and drain the excess water.
2. Bring the measured amount of grain and liquid (either vegetable stock or water) to a boil. You can add a pinch of sea salt.
3. Cover with a tight-fitting lid, lower the heat to low, and simmer for the recommended time. Because the grain is being steamed, do not lift the lid until the grain is finished cooking.

The following chart will give you an approximate cooking time and yield of some of the more popular grains. Cooking times may vary depending upon altitude and stove cooking temperatures. The grain is generally finished cooking when it is chewy and all of the liquid is absorbed.

Many grains can be prepared in less than thirty minutes. If you wish to turn a recipe in the book into a thirty-minute meal, begin cooking the grain before starting a recipe, and the grain will typically be finished by the time you are done preparing the other dishes.

Cooking Beans and Legumes

Beans and legumes are a high-fiber, low-calorie, low-fat, low-sodium, and cholesterol-free food. They are also relatively high in protein, amino acids, vitamins, and minerals. If you have time to soak and prepare a pot of beans, you will save on the packaging of the canned products.

Before you cook legumes, it is recommended to clean them thoroughly, rinse them well, and soak them overnight. This improves their digestibility and reduces gas. Other methods for improving digestibility include adding some fennel seeds, a handful of brown rice, or a few strips of the sea vegetable kombu to the legumes while cooking. If you do not have time to soak the beans overnight, a quick method to soften them is to bring the beans plus water four times their volume to a boil, remove from the heat, cover, and allow to sit for a few hours.

Grain Cooking Chart				
Grain	Liquid/cup of grain	Approx. cooking time (minutes)	Approx. yield (cups)	Comments
Amaranth	2½	25	2½	Ancient grain of Aztecs, higher in protein and nutrients than most grains
Barley, pearled	3	45	3½	Good in soups and stews
Buckwheat	2	15	2½	Hearty, nutty flavor. When toasted it's called kasha. Can be used as a breakfast cereal, and comes in several grinds, from fine to coarse.
Couscous	1½	15	1½	A North African staple made from ground semolina
Millet	2½	20	3	A highly nutritious, gluten-free grain with origins in ancient China. Used in casseroles, stews, and cereals, or on its own as a side dish.
Oats, Steel cut	3	30–40	3	A versatile grain that is popular as a cereal and for baking. Steel cut oats are oat groats that have been cut into smaller pieces.
Oats, Rolled	3	10	3	Oat groats that have been steamed and rolled into flakes for quicker cooking
Oats, Quick	2	5	2	Rolled oats that have been cut into smaller pieces for even quicker cooking
Polenta	3	10	3	A type of cornmeal used in Italian cooking

continues

Grain Cooking Chart *continued*

Grain	Liquid/cup of grain	Approx. cooking time (minutes)	Approx. yield (cups)	Comments
Quinoa	2	20	2½	Ancient grain of the Incans—high in protein and many nutrients; has a delicate, nutty flavor.
Rice, Brown Basmati	2	35–40	2¼	Rice has a high nutrient content and is a staple in many of the world's cultures. Basmati rice has a nutty flavor and is used in Indian cooking.
Rice, White Basmati	1½	20	2	A quick-cooking rice with a nice presentation
Rice, Brown long-grain	2	45	3	Stays fluffy and separated after cooking. Great for pilafs and stir-fries.
Rice, Brown, short-grain	2	45	3	A popular rice with full flavor. After cooking, grains are soft and stick together. Great for nori rolls and as a side dish.
Rice, Wild	3	60	4	A festive rice, popular in holiday dishes
Spelt Berries	3½	90	3	Spelt is an ancient form of wheat. Boil for use in salads.
Teff	3	20	1½	From Ethiopia, the smallest grain in the world. It is the main ingredient for injera flatbread.
Wheat, Bulgur	2	15	2½	Wheat is a primary bread grain. Bulgur is used in Middle Eastern dishes such as tabbouleh.
Wheat, Cracked	2	25	2½	Cracked wheat may be used as a cereal.

After soaking the legumes or boiling them in this way, discard the soak water, add the measured amount of vegetable stock or water to a thick-bottomed pot, bring to a boil, cover, reduce the heat to a simmer, and cook until tender. The times in the following chart are for cooking dried legumes.

Do not add salt to the cooking liquid; it can make the legumes tough. Legumes are done cooking when they are tender but not mushy. They should retain their original shape.

Note: These times are for cooking dried beans. Please reduce cooking time by 25 percent if the beans have been soaked.

Dried Bean Cooking Chart				
Legume	Liquid/cup of legume	Approx. cooking time	Approx. yield (cups)	Comments
Adzuki Beans	3¼	45 mins	3	Tender red bean used in Japanese and macrobiotic cooking
Anasazi Beans	3	2 hrs	2	Means "the Ancient Ones" in Navajo language; sweeter and meatier than most beans
Black Beans (Turtle Beans)	4	1¼ hrs	2½	Good in Spanish, South American, and Caribbean dishes
Black-Eyed Peas	4	1¼ hrs	2	A staple of the American South
Garbanzo Beans (Chickpeas)	4	3–4 hrs	2	Used in Middle Eastern and Indian dishes
Great Northern Beans	4	1½ hrs	2	Beautiful, large white bean
Kidney Beans	4	1½ hrs	2	Medium-size red beans; most popular bean in the United States, also used in Mexican cooking
Lentils Green Red	 3 3	 45 mins 25 min	 2¼ 2¼	Come in green, red, and French varieties. A member of the pea family, used in Indian dhal dishes and soups.

continues

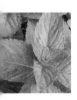

Dried Bean Cooking Chart *continued*				
Legume	Liquid/cup of legume	Approx. cooking time	Approx. yield (cups)	Comments
Lima Beans,	3	1½ hrs	1¼	White bean with a distinctive
Baby Limas	3	1½ hrs	1¾	flavor; high in nutrients
Mung Beans	3	45 mins	2¼	Grown in India and Asia; used in Indian dhal dishes. May be soaked and sprouted and used fresh in soups and salads (bean sprouts).
Navy Beans (White Beans)	4	2½ hrs	2	A hearty bean used in soups, stews, and cold salads
Pinto Beans	4	2½ hrs	2	Used in Mexican and Southwestern cooking. Used in soups and as refried beans in burritos.
Split Peas	3	45 mins	2¼	Come in yellow and green varieties; they do not need to be soaked. Used in soups and Indian dhals.

Toasting Spices, Nuts, and Seeds

Toasting is another method to bring out a deeper flavor of ingredients. There are two methods we commonly use. Toasting can be done in a dry sauté pan. For this method, place the food in a pan, turn the heat to high, and cook until the item turns golden brown, stirring constantly. This method is good for spices, grains, and small quantities of nuts or seeds. Another method involves preheating an oven to 350°F. Place the food on a dry baking sheet and leave in the oven until golden brown, stirring occasionally and being mindful to avoid burning. This method is best for nuts, seeds, and shredded coconut. Nuts become crunchier after cooling down. As mentioned earlier, if you have more time, you can enhance the flavor even more by roasting at lower temperatures for longer periods of time. Nuts, for instance, roasted at 200°F for 45 minutes, have a richer, toastier flavor than if roasted at a high temperature for a shorter period of time.

Working with Tofu

Tofu is sold in a number of different forms, including extra-firm, firm, medium, soft, and silken. Each different form lends itself to a particular type of food preparation. The recipes will describe which form of tofu is required for the dish.

- The silken style may be blended and used to replace dairy products in puddings, frostings, dressings, creamy soups, and sauces.
- The soft type may be used cubed in soups or pureed in sauces, spreads, or dips.
- The medium and firm styles may be scrambled, grated in casseroles, or cubed in stir-fries.
- The extra-firm style may be grilled or baked as cutlets, or it may be cubed and roasted. It may also be steamed and used in steamed veggie dishes.

Leftover tofu should be rinsed and covered with water in a glass container in the refrigerator. Changing water daily is recommended. Use within four days. Firm and extra-firm tofu may be frozen for up to three months. Frozen tofu, once defrosted, has a spongy texture that absorbs marinades more than tofu that has not been frozen.

To make tofu cutlets: Slice a one-pound block of extra-firm tofu into thirds or fourths. If you wish, you can then cut these cutlets in half to yield six or eight cutlets per pound. You can also cut the tofu diagonally to create triangle-shaped cutlets. Cutlets can be marinated and then roasted or grilled.

To make tofu cubes: To make medium-size cubes, slice the tofu as you would for three or four cutlets. Then make four cuts along the length and three cuts along the width of the tofu. You can make the cubes larger or smaller by altering the number of cuts.

Working with Tempeh

Tempeh needs to be thoroughly cooked before consuming. It is typically available in an eight-ounce package. Several varieties come in a thick, square block. Others come as a thinner rectangle. Some recommend steaming the tempeh for ten minutes before using in dishes, to remove the bitterness. Store leftover tempeh in a sealed glass container in the refrigerator for up to three days.

To make tempeh cutlets: You can slice the square block in half to create a thinner block and then cut it in half or into triangles. The longer block may also be sliced into thinner cutlets. These cutlets may then be cut into cubes.

Roasting Tofu and Tempeh:

Tofu and tempeh cubes can be marinated, roasted, and then stored for a couple of days in a glass container in the refrigerator to be used in salads, stir-fries, or on their own as a snack.

To roast tofu and tempeh cutlets and cubes, follow these simple steps:

1. Preheat the oven or toaster oven to 350°F. Cut the tofu or tempeh into cutlets or cubes as mentioned above.
2. Place them in a marinade of your choosing (see page 21). Allow them to sit for at least 5 minutes and up to overnight. If marinating overnight, store in an airtight container in the refrigerator.
3. Place on a well-oiled baking sheet or casserole dish. Roast until golden brown, approximately 20 minutes, stirring the cubes occasionally to ensure even cooking. If making cutlets, you can flip them after 10 minutes. Try a convection oven or use a broil setting, for a crispier crust.

We prefer to use the toaster oven for small quantities of up to one pound of tofu or tempeh. One pound of tofu or tempeh conveniently fits in the baking tray. Be aware that food tends to cook faster in a toaster oven than a regular oven. Depending on the toaster, you can typically roast the tofu or tempeh in 15 minutes instead of 20.

Grilling

Consider grilling tempeh and tofu cutlets, as well as many vegetables and fruits such as Portobello mushrooms, corn, onions, baby bok choy, bell peppers, asparagus, zucchini, coconut meat, pineapple slices, or eggplant. If you wish for added flavor, place the food in a marinade before grilling from a few minutes to overnight (see page 21). Baste or brush with oil, brushing occasionally and grilling until char marks appear and the item is heated thoroughly, flipping it periodically. If using a gas grill, avoid placing the items over a direct flame.

Another grilling option is to use a stove-top grill. Kitchen supply stores sell cast-iron and nonstick pans that are flat, straddle two burners, and have a griddle on one side and a grooved side for grilling. The flavor is similar and you get the fancy char marks without having to fuss with (or own) a grill.

Juicing

Fresh organic juices are an important part of a healthy lifestyle. Juicing makes the nutrients in fruits and vegetables easier to assimilate. Enjoy juices on their own or in smoothies, live soups, sauces, and dressings as a convenient way to meet the recommended daily allowance of five to nine servings of fruits and vegetables.

Some juicy tips to consider:

- Use fresh organic fruits and vegetables whenever possible.
- 1 pound of produce yields approximately 8 ounces of juice.
- It is recommended to drink juices within 20 minutes of juicing, to receive the maximum nutritional benefit.
- It's best not to mix fruits and vegetables in the same juice. Sometimes we do add a little apple to sweeten a vegetable juice, or lemon to our green juices.
- For vegetable juices, use carrots as the base and then experiment with different quantities and types of veggies.
- Some like to add water to dilute straight fruit juices or even sweet vegetable juices, such as straight carrot, to balance the effect on blood sugar levels.
- Add other ingredients to enhance the flavor and nutritional quality of your juices, blending them in. Try ground flaxseeds, or supplements such as spirulina and maca powder.

Cracking a Coconut

Known as the "tree of life" or *niu* in Hawaiian, the coconut palm (*Cocos nucifera*) has been a staple in tropical climates for centuries. Young coconuts, at about six months of age, have a jellylike center with a texture similar to a melon, which can be scooped out of their shell with a spoon. It has a fresh, fruity, almost nutty flavor, not overly sweet. As the coconut ages, this jelly becomes the meat. The older the coconut, the drier the meat, until it is like the dark brown coconut you find in the market.

The jelly and juice of young coconuts can be consumed straight from the shell, whereas the flesh of more mature coconuts is blended to make coconut cream and milk. (The liquid inside the center of the coconut is coconut water, not coconut milk.) Try to locate young coconuts at Asian or Latin markets.

Cutting a coconut isn't difficult, but you should be very careful. Place the coconut on its side on a sturdy cutting board or the ground, and hold the bottom of the coconut. Using a heavy cleaver or machete, carefully give it a whack about 1½ inches below the pointed end. This should cut into the hard shell. If not, you can give it another light whack, being careful not to spill the water. Place the coconut over a bowl or a quart-size mason jar and drain out the liquid, which can be stored in a glass jar in the refrigerator for two to three days. If pieces of the shell fell into the water, strain them out. Once the liquid is removed, you can use the knife to carefully pry off the remainder of the top for easy removal of the meat.

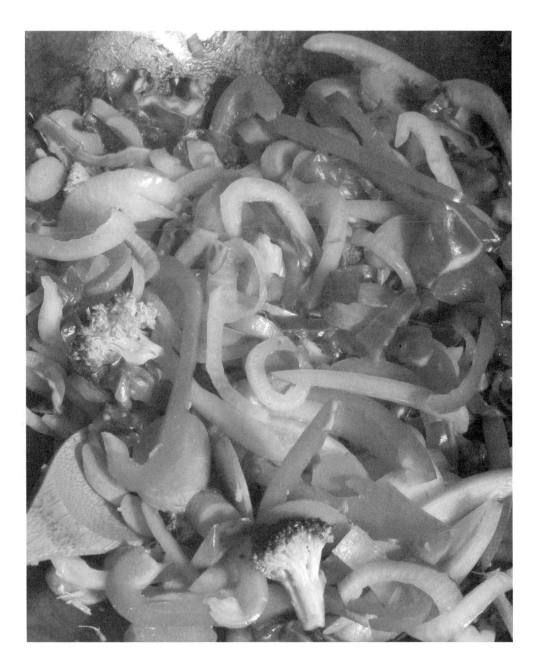

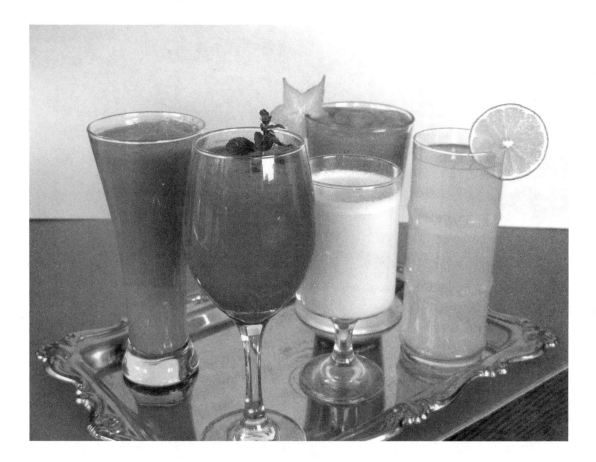

CHAPTER 3

The Lighter Side of Life—Smoothies & Satiating Beverages

D on't let this chapter's position at the beginning of the book trick you into thinking these beverages are only for morning. Often a meal unto themselves, beverages can provide an abundance of nutrition and satisfaction—for breakfast, lunch, or dinner.

Here we offer a selection of tantalizing juices, smoothies, and elixirs. A fresh juice is preferable to a salty or sugary snack anytime. Limeade quenches your thirst and your sweet tooth on a hot sunny day. An almond butter smoothie can easily masquerade as a dessert. So simple, fast, and a joy to create! We also introduce a recipe for nut and seed milk—an essential for raw food preparation.

Being prepared for that emergency smoothie is easy once you get the hang of it. Keep some dates soaking in water in a glass container in the refrigerator. These will last up to a week. Keep whole peeled bananas in an airtight plastic bag or glass container in the freezer. You can also blend fresh fruit, such as papayas, mangoes, strawberries, and peaches, into a puree, pour into ice cube trays, and freeze. Use in smoothies or to add an interesting flavor to juices.

A good drink can take the place of an appetizer when you are having guests. Picture the scene. You are still working on the food when your guests arrive early and hungry now! Rather than hurrying out a plate of sliced watermelon, you throw that same watermelon in the blender with a little rose water and suddenly you are the brilliant culinary mastermind that saved the day. You genius, you! And everyone still has room for the dinner you are making.

A couple of tips to get the most out of your beverages:

- Always drink fresh juice within twenty minutes, for optimal flavor and nutrition.
- For all juice recipes, yields are approximate and will vary depending on the produce and the strength of your juicer.
- Check out the juicing section in chapter 2 for more tips and tricks on the art of juicing.

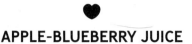

APPLE-BLUEBERRY JUICE

Berries aren't quite juicy enough to enjoy an entire glass by themselves. Luckily, they create sweet harmony with so many other fruits.

MAKES APPROXIMATELY TWO 12-OUNCE SERVINGS

1 pound blueberries (about 3 cups)
1 (1- to 2-inch) piece fresh ginger (optional)
4 medium-size apples, quartered

1. Run all of the ingredients through a juicer and enjoy in the bright sunshine!
2. You may want to start with the berries, then the ginger, and finish off with the apples, to clean all of the berry and ginger juice from the juicer.

Variations
- Replace the blueberries with an equal amount of other berries, such as raspberries, blackberries, or strawberries. Or try other fruits, such as cherries or grapes.
- Replace all or some of the apple with pear or an equal amount of pineapple.

Superfoods for Health

All fresh fruits contain antioxidants, but berries really take the cake! In particular, blueberries are a treasure trove of these cell-protecting antioxidants.

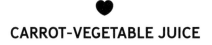

CARROT-VEGETABLE JUICE

This classic vegetable juice, high in vitamins C and A, is actually quite sweet, so you may wish to dilute it with a bit of water. You can also try mixing in a tablespoon of ground flaxseeds per glass to balance out the sweetness and the effect on blood sugar levels. If the ginger is organic and the skin is thin, you don't need to peel it.

MAKES APPROXIMATELY TWO 10-OUNCE SERVINGS

Several sprigs of parsley	½ medium beet
6 stalks celery	10 medium-size carrots
1 (1½-inch) piece fresh ginger	

1. Put all of the ingredients through a juicer, in the order listed above, and enjoy. Putting the least juicy stuff through first and ending with the juiciest is an effective way to get all of the goods into your cup.
2. Strain if you wish for a smoother, albeit less nutritious beverage. If you are not able to drink immediately, store in a tightly sealed glass jar in the refrigerator. You can increase the amount of parsley according to your taste, up to about one ounce.

Variations

- Countless variations are possible. Using carrots as a base, add your favorite veggies and herbs, such as cabbage, tomato, lettuce, bell pepper, kale, beet greens, or cilantro in quantities that suit your fancy.
- Try leaving out all of the veggies except the carrots and blending with 1 cup of almond milk (page 42) and ½ teaspoon of nutmeg, for **Jamaican carrot juice**.

Quicker and Easier

Straight carrot juice is one of the best ways to introduce kids to vegetable juices. You can slowly add other veggies once they are accustomed to the carrot juice on its own. Adding a small amount of apple makes the juice even more kid-friendly.

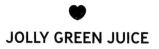

JOLLY GREEN JUICE

Get your green on with this nutritious beverage that makes a refreshing elixir first thing in the morning or anytime you wish to put a little zip into your day. You can adjust the apple quantity to your desired sweetness.

MAKES APPROXIMATELY TWO 10-OUNCE SERVINGS

6 large leaves kale

6 stalks celery

2 large cucumbers

1 small lemon, peeled

2 large apples, quartered

1. Cut the cucumbers, apples, and lemon so that they will fit through the juicer.
2. Run all of the ingredients through a juicer, in the order listed above, and enjoy. Strain if desired.

Variations

- Replace the kale with Swiss chard or your favorite dark leafy green.
- Add a ½-inch piece of fresh ginger and/or a clove of garlic.
- Try replacing the apple with pineapple or pear.

Superfoods for Health

Green juices and smoothies are perhaps the most nutritious way to get your daily supply of dark leafy greens—revered for their potent antioxidant levels, and powerhouse of minerals and vitamins. The green comes from the high quantities of chlorophyll, which helps the plants convert energy from the light of the sun.

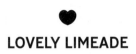

LOVELY LIMEADE

Put limes to good use with this satisfying alternative to traditional lemonade. Made with coconut water and vanilla, it's the ultimate tropical refresher.

MAKES TWO 14-OUNCE SERVINGS

Seeds from ½ vanilla bean, or
2 teaspoons vanilla extract (optional)

½ cup freshly squeezed lime juice

2½ cups coconut water or water

¼ cup + 2 tablespoons agave nectar or
organic cane sugar, or to taste

Mint leaves and lime wedges
(optional)

1. If using the seeds of the vanilla bean, blend them well with the lime juice, coconut water, and agave nectar.
2. Otherwise, simply stir all of the ingredients well in a pitcher. Garnish the glasses with mint leaves and lime wedges, if desired.

Variations

- For lemonade, replace limes with . . . you guessed it . . . lemons.
- For lime-gingerade, add a ¼- to ½-inch piece of fresh ginger—blend and strain before serving.
- For pink limeade, add a very small sliver of beet before blending. A little goes a long way with beets.
- For lavender-rose limeade, add 1 teaspoon of lavender flowers and 1 tablespoon of rose water before blending. Strain before serving.

CHERRY-VANILLA SPRITZER

This homemade brew is perfect for when you are looking for something a bit jazzier than a fruit juice. There are many pluses to this recipe: it allows you to control the amount of sweetness of your beverage; it also calls for numerous variations; and, as an added bonus, these syrups can also be used on the "Buttermilk" Pancakes (page 66), Waffles (page 270), or French Toast (page 71).

MAKES FOUR 12-OUNCE SERVINGS

10 ounces frozen cherries, thawed (If you don't have time to defrost the cherries, you may need to add a bit of water to get things going in the blender.)

¾ cup agave nectar, pure maple syrup, or organic sugar, or to taste

2 tablespoons vanilla extract, or the seeds of 1 vanilla bean

48 ounces sparkling water (6 cups)

Fresh cherries (optional)

Orange slices (optional)

1. For the syrup, place cherries, agave nectar, and vanilla in a blender and blend until smooth.
2. Place 5 to 6 tablespoons of the syrup in a large glass with ½ cup of the sparkling water. Stir well until the syrup is dissolved. Add another 1 cup of sparkling water and gently stir. Use more or less syrup to desired sweetness. Garnish with a fresh cherry and/or orange slice, if using. Repeat this step with additional glasses to make the other three servings.

Variations

- Replace the frozen berries with 2 cups of fresh berries. If using a granulated sugar, you may need to add ¼ to ½ cup of water to reach a syrupy consistency.
- Try with other berries, such as strawberries. If you use raspberries, pour the syrup through a fine-mesh strainer after blending to remove the seeds.
- Expand your repertoire by experimenting with other fruits, such as peach, pineapple, mango, and papaya.
- If you want to enjoy a unique syrup for pancakes, waffles, or French toast, simply follow step 1.

INDIAN CHAI LATTE

Chai in India comes in almost as many varieties as curry, so the elusive "authentic" Indian chai remains a matter of taste. This thick, spicy, and mildly sweet recipe uses a very simplified method with fantastic results.

MAKES FOUR 12-OUNCE SERVINGS

¼ cup cardamom pods

⅓ cup (2- to 3-inch-long) cinnamon sticks

½ cup fresh ginger, chopped small

1 teaspoon whole black peppercorns

1 teaspoon whole cloves

6 cups rice milk (see Tips and Tricks)

2 tea bags black tea (optional), such as harmutty or a breakfast tea,
or 1½ teaspoons of loose leaf tea

2 tablespoons pure maple syrup or ¼ cup brown rice syrup

1. Place the cardamom pods and cinnamon sticks in a blender and pulse-chop two or three times to break them up a bit. Don't blend them into a powder. Place them in a pot with the ginger, peppercorns, cloves, and rice milk. Bring the mixture to a boil over low heat, and simmer for 10 to 15 minutes.
2. Turn off the heat and, if desired, add the tea, and steep for 3 to 5 minutes (depending upon the tea). Strain the liquid through a fine-mesh strainer and return to the pot over low heat.
3. Add the maple syrup and whisk. Serve immediately.

Tips and Tricks

For this recipe we recommend using rice milk over soy or other milks because it won't thicken as much as it cooks. If you are using another milk, you may want to dilute the milk with water by one quarter to one half, depending on the thickness of your choice of milk.

Variations

- Try using allspice, anise, coriander, and nutmeg along with, or instead of, some of the spices listed here.
- Try substituting green tea, such as gunpowder, for the black tea. Also try using red teas such as rooibos, vanilla rooibos, or African honeybush tea. You can even substitute more robust teas such as Earl Grey, smoky Russian caravan, or Mate.

If You Have More Time

If you wish to use a fresh nut milk from page 42, replace the 6 cups of rice milk with 4 cups of water, and follow all of the other directions. To serve, combine ⅓ cup of nut milk and ⅔ cup of chai. Fresh walnut milk is a stellar choice. Letting the walnuts soak for a day or two before making the milk releases most of their bitter tannins, leaving a sweet nutty flavor instead.

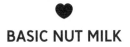

BASIC NUT MILK

A revolutionary and certified cow-free way to enjoy milk, this is a favorite in our home and a must-have for raw food preparation. Try it with almonds, macadamia nuts, sesame seeds, Brazil nuts, or any of the seeds and nuts in the chart on page 43. Use this base recipe to create countless varieties of nut and seed milks. Each combination will provide its own unique flavor. Experiment with macadamia–pine nut, almond–hemp seed, or walnut-cashew milk. Partake of this milk in all recipes that call for milk or on its own as a refreshing beverage.

MAKES 1 QUART

1 cup shelled nut or seeds

4 cups water

1. Rinse the nuts well and drain. If you have more time, as well as for best results, see the chart on the next page for recommended soak times.
2. Place the nuts in a blender with the water and blend on high speed for 30 seconds or until creamy.
3. Strain the milk through a fine-mesh strainer, cheesecloth, or fine-mesh bag. If using a fine-mesh strainer, use a spoon or rubber spatula to swirl the nut meal around, which allows the milk to drain faster.
4. If desired, sweeten with agave nectar or maple syrup to taste.

Variation
- This recipe also works for rice milk. Just follow the ratios, using uncooked brown rice and water. It's a convenient way to save on packaging; it's fresh and tastes better!

Nut, seed, and rice milks will last for 3 to 4 days when stored in an airtight glass jar in the refrigerator.

If You Have More Time

Soaking Chart

For increased nutritional value and to enhance diges-
tion, rinse nuts or seeds well and place them in a bowl
or jar with water in a ratio of one part nuts/
seeds to three or four parts water. Allow them to
sit for the recommended time, covered, at room temperature, before draining, rinsing, and using in recipes.

Nut/Seed	Soak Time in hours
Almonds	4 to 6
Brazil nuts	4 to 6
Cashews	1 to 2
Hazelnuts	4 to 6
Macadamia nuts	1 to 2
Pecans	4 to 6
Pine nuts	1 to 2
Pumpkin seeds	1 to 4
Sesame seeds	1 to 4
Sunflower seeds	1 to 4
Walnuts	4 to 6

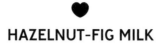

HAZELNUT-FIG MILK

This is just one of many ways you can create unique creamy nut milks, using the basic recipe. The fig and hazelnut combo is especially tasty. Try experimenting with different varieties of figs and nuts. Vary the amount of figs or add agave nectar to enhance sweetness.

MAKES 1 QUART

6 dried figs
4 cups water
1 cup hazelnuts

1. Place the figs in a bowl with 4 cups of water for 15 minutes. Place the hazelnuts in another bowl with a few cups of water for 15 minutes.
2. Drain the hazelnuts, rinse well, and place in the blender. Add the fig soak water, but not the figs, to a blender with the hazelnuts and blend well. Pour this mixture through a fine-mesh strainer, cheesecloth, or fine-mesh bag, saving the liquid in a bowl and discarding any hazelnut meal left in the strainer. If using a fine-mesh strainer, use a spoon to swirl the meal around, which allows the milk to drain faster.
3. Return ½ to 1 cup of the milk to the blender and blend with the figs until creamy. Add the remaining milk, blend, and enjoy.

Variations
- Add 3 tablespoons of raw cacao nibs or powder and/or 1 teaspoon of maca powder to the finished product and reblend.
- Replace the hazelnuts and figs with your favorite nuts, seeds, and dried fruits. Some combinations to consider include Brazil nut–apricot milk, hemp-date milk, sunflower-raisin milk, or carob-mint-almond milk.

Quicker and Easier

A highly refreshing beverage consists of placing some dried figs in a mason jar or water bottle and filling it with water. Over time, the water takes on a fig flavor. Bring along on a hike, and when you are finished drinking the water, you can feast on the plump figs. The fig water will last for 1 day if left unrefrigerated, and for 3 days if stored in the refrigerator.

♥
WATERMELON COOLER

It is hard to improve upon simple watermelon slices. But give this drink or any of its variations a whirl and you, too, will soon be a drinkable watermelon convert. Little else can be so refreshing! Depending on how sweet your watermelon is, you may wish to add a little agave nectar as well. Use a cold, refrigerated watermelon and/or frosted glasses if you desire to serve cold drinks immediately.

MAKES FOUR 10-OUNCE SERVINGS

6 cups scooped watermelon, seeded

2 tablespoons freshly squeezed lime juice

¼ cup mint leaves, lightly packed

Agave nectar, to taste, if necessary

1. Blend everything together until the mint leaves are well ground up.
2. Serve immediately or refrigerate to chill.

Variations
- For a plain watermelon slushie, just use the above recipe minus all of the ingredients except the watermelon, adding the agave nectar to taste.
- Another pretty party presentation is to add 1 tablespoon of food-grade rose water to a full blender of watermelon for a delicate floral drink. Try sprinkling with culinary-safe rosebuds, too!
- For a berry-melon version, use one 10-ounce package of frozen strawberries or raspberries and fill the rest of the blender with watermelon. Blend and add agave nectar as necessary. Some lime or lemon juice will go beautifully with this as well (start with 2 tablespoons).

Tips and Tricks

A good trick for keeping this beverage cold at parties is to freeze some of the mixture in an ice cube tray and serve the cubes with the drink, or add some cubes and reblend before serving.

Quicker and Easier

Herbal and green teas make a refreshing beverage. To conserve on packaging, try using loose teas and herbs, such as chamomile, mint, or yerba mate in bulk and using a tea ball rather than purchasing individually packaged teas. Bagged teas are quite convenient to have in a pinch and there is a wide range of brands to choose from; Yogi Tea, Tazo, the Republic of Tea, and Numi put out superior products. Whatever brand or style you choose, it's easy to whip up a quick drink. Just add ice and a sprig of mint to create an herbal iced tea du jour.

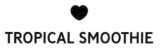

TROPICAL SMOOTHIE

Vanilla is one of our all-time fave smoothie ingredients. If coconut butter is not readily available to you, this smoothie rocks without it. And it is a much better way to start the day than with the usual heavier starchy carbs.

MAKES FOUR 10-OUNCE SERVINGS

1½ cups mango, peeled and cubed

1½ cups pineapple, skin and core removed, cubed

2 large bananas, fresh or frozen

1 cup freshly squeezed orange juice

½ teaspoon vanilla extract, preferably alcohol-free

1 to 2 tablespoons coconut butter (optional)

1. Blend all of the ingredients together until smooth.
2. Serve immediately or refrigerate for up to 24 hours in an airtight glass jar.

Variations

- You can substitute store-bought orange juice for the fresh OJ if you prefer. Apple juice is another good alternative, but these days health food stores carry a huge variety of interesting juice combinations you can play with.
- Try using fresh or frozen berries, peaches, pears, apples, or pomegranate.

Quicker and Easier

Place the skin and core of the pineapple in a jar, fill with water, and refrigerate. This creates a subtly sweet water that can be used in smoothies or enjoyed on its own. Toss in a couple of cinnamon sticks and aniseeds for added flavor. Enjoy within 3 days for maximum freshness.

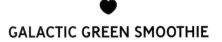

GALACTIC GREEN SMOOTHIE

Yummy smoothies are an effortless way to get some high-quality raw greens into your system. Greens are filled with minerals and other nutrients that our bodies thrive on. And greens make your skin glow, too, so drink up for your health and enjoy the side effects! You may wish to start with a smaller quantity of greens while you grow accustomed to the concept. Don't knock it 'til you've tried it, though. If you do not have access to papayas, replace them with an equal amount of pineapple.

MAKES TWO 16-OUNCE SERVINGS

4 pitted dates (preferably Medjool)

¾ cup apple juice

1 large banana (about 1 cup sliced)

1 medium-size papaya, seeded (about 2 cups flesh) (see Tips and Tricks)

¼ cup cashews or macadamia nuts

3 cups kale leaves, lightly packed

1. If you do not have Medjool dates, which are moister than other dates, you may want to first blend the dates and apple juice together to puree them. Give it a good 30 seconds or so. (You can also use soaked dates if you followed our suggestion to have soaked dates on hand in the fridge.)
2. Otherwise, blend all of the ingredients, starting on low speed and working your way up to high speed until smooth.

Tips and Tricks

Papayas range from the size of a pear to the size of a watermelon. Depending on the season, you'll see different varieties of papayas in many shapes and sizes (any of which will work in this recipe). Try to follow closely to the recipe measurement of 2 cups of the scooped out flesh to get the right amount and consistency. Also, be sure not to get ANY of the seeds in the smoothie. Even one can make the whole batch taste peppery.

Variations

- Substitute pineapple juice, coconut nectar, or pear juice for the apple juice. Or try any of your favorite juices that you think will match.
- Substitute any kind of nonbitter lettuce such as green-leaf, red-leaf, or butter-head lettuce for the kale.
- Adding several mint leaves will create a fresh taste.
- Substituting peanut butter or almond butter for the cashews offers a different, equally rich and delightful taste.

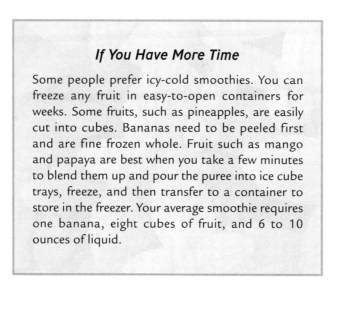

If You Have More Time

Some people prefer icy-cold smoothies. You can freeze any fruit in easy-to-open containers for weeks. Some fruits, such as pineapples, are easily cut into cubes. Bananas need to be peeled first and are fine frozen whole. Fruit such as mango and papaya are best when you take a few minutes to blend them up and pour the puree into ice cube trays, freeze, and then transfer to a container to store in the freezer. Your average smoothie requires one banana, eight cubes of fruit, and 6 to 10 ounces of liquid.

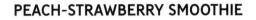

PEACH-STRAWBERRY SMOOTHIE

Breakfast in a glass is the way to go on busy mornings. Consider this nature's bounty in a made-for-the-road package. You can find organic frozen strawberries and peaches in 10-ounce bags at health food stores. If you use fresh peaches and/or strawberries rather than frozen for this beverage, you won't need to use so much apple juice. Start with one cup instead of two. If you don't have any frozen bananas on hand, fresh will do. Do not thaw the fruit before blending.

MAKES TWO 16-OUNCE SERVINGS

2 frozen bananas

5 ounces frozen strawberries (about 1 heaping cup)

5 ounces frozen peaches (about 1 heaping cup)

2 cups apple juice

1. Blend all of the ingredients together on high speed until smooth. You may need to add a little more apple juice.
2. Go slowly—you can always add more but you can't take it away.

Variations

- Try substituting soy milk, pineapple juice, or your favorite juice for the apple juice.
- Try adding 1 teaspoon of freshly squeezed lime juice for a zestier flavor.
- Add ½ teaspoon of vanilla extract for a creamier flavor.

Superfoods for Health

Enhance the power of your smoothies with some high-nutrition add-ons. Some of our favorites include spirulina, ground flaxseeds, maca powder, cacao nibs, or goji berries. We sometimes enjoy adding other supplements such as New Greens or Berry Fusion from Pure Prescriptions. You can also add açaí, the South American superberry that can be purchased frozen in the United States. It's considered to have the most antioxidants of any fruit. Follow the manufacturer's suggested serving size or just add to your heart's content.

ALMOND BUTTER SMOOTHIE

Luscious and sweet and so good to eat, this smoothie is great when there isn't much fruit in season. It very much helps if the bananas are frozen but it isn't absolutely necessary. When made with freshly grated nutmeg, this smoothie becomes habit forming.

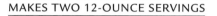

MAKES TWO 12-OUNCE SERVINGS

4 pitted dates	¼ teaspoon ground cinnamon
2 medium-size frozen bananas	Pinch of grated nutmeg (optional)
6 tablespoons roasted almond butter	1½ cups rice milk

1. Soak the dates in water to cover for 20 minutes and strain.
2. Blend the dates with the remaining ingredients until harmony on earth prevails or until a thick, uniform consistency is reached, about 1 minute.

Variations

- Adding 1 tablespoon of cacao nibs, carob powder, or unsweetened cocoa powder to this smoothie absolutely cannot hurt.
- Substituting almond milk (see page 42) for the rice milk will move this into the ultradecadent range.
- If you don't have dates, substitute 1 to 2 tablespoons of agave nectar or maple syrup and another ½ banana for thickness.
- ♥ For a raw version, use homemade Nut Milk (page 42) and raw almond butter.

Quicker and Easier

All these beverages have the benefits of being tasty **and** healthy and are good pick-me-ups for any occasion. But let's not forgot about the ultimate beverage: good clean water. Spice up your glass of water with a few lemon or lime wedges. Herbal waters are also a refreshing change. Place a stalk of rosemary, a few sprigs of cilantro, or several basil leaves in a mason jar with water (plus ice if you like). Other flavors can be created with ginger slices, chamomile tea flowers, fresh mint, fresh ginger flowers, organic mini roses from your garden . . . the list goes on and on.

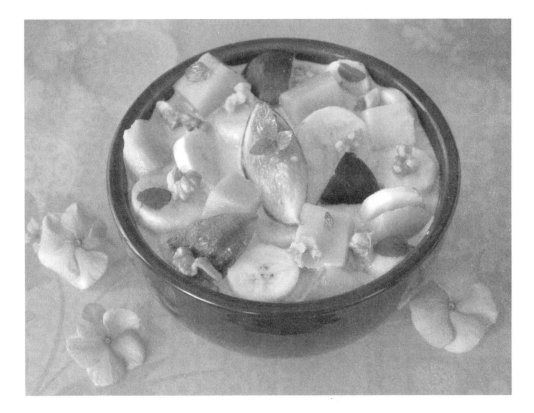

CHAPTER 4

The Morning Meal—
Breakfast & Brunch

Wake up, smile, and start the day the vegan way with these healthful and satisfying morning recipes. Many say that breakfast is the most important meal, that it sets the tone for the rest of the day. This chapter provides a wide range of options for you to enjoy, from a simple multigrain hot cereal to a gourmet meal that will satisfy the hungriest among us. If you're one of the many people who find that a live breakfast is the most energizing way to begin the day, you'll find plenty of raw recipes to whet your appetite here.

Brunch is an art form unto itself. It's an excuse to eat waaay more than you might at breakfast because you are getting in two meals' worth of food at one sitting. And since none of these recipes take more than thirty minutes to complete, you'll have ample time to relax and enjoy. Whether it's Tofu Scramble, Tempeh Bacon, and Seasoned Spuds, or crepes, French toast, and pancakes, these recipes are sure to please. So invite your friends over and get your brunch on!

♥

WALNUT-SPRINKLED FRUIT BOWL

The variations of fruits and nuts you may use for this dish are limited only by what is available to you. Consider this recipe a starting point. The idea is that a bowl of fresh fruit, sprinkled with some chopped nuts and covered in your favorite kind of milk, is a lovely and refreshing breakfast. We highly recommend using fresh almond milk (see page 42).

SERVES 2

1 large mango, peeled and cubed (see Tips and Tricks)

2 large figs, chopped

2 medium-size bananas, sliced

¼ cup walnuts, chopped

1 cup nondairy milk of choice

1. Prepare all of the fruits and divide them evenly between two bowls.
2. Sprinkle each bowl with the walnuts and cover with ½ cup of the nondairy milk. Enjoy!

Tips and Tricks

The easiest way to cube a mango: Slice off the stem end. Hold the mango with the stem end flat on the cutting board and turn it so that you can slice off the narrower sides, avoiding the seed but coming as close to it as possible. Then slice the thin strips off either side of the seed. Take the two larger pieces and score a checkerboard into the fruit with your knife. Use a spoon to scoop out the cubes. Then score the narrow strips and scoop out the cubes. We always carve whatever fruit we can off of the seed as well.

Quicker and Easier

For a quick breakfast treat, slice a papaya in half and scoop out the seeds. Enjoy with a splash of freshly squeezed lime juice and a pinch of chile powder for a bold combination of sweet, tangy, and spicy. You can also add some fresh berries and sliced banana for a fruit salad on the go. (The lime and chile combo also goes well with pineapple slices).

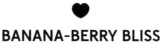

BANANA-BERRY BLISS

This is another dish that's at the height of simplicity and bursting with flavor and color. Summer mornings when berries are abundant, this is the dish for you. Vary the fruits, or swap the macadamia nuts for cashews in the cream, to create different flavors. Make a double batch of the cream and use it for Banana Pudding (page 255) or Live Fruit Parfait (page 261).

SERVES 4

4 small bananas, sliced

4 cups blueberries, raspberries, blackberries, sliced strawberries, or a combination of all

1 recipe Crème de la Crème

Mint leaves

Crème de la Crème

(yields 2¼ cups)

1 cup macadamia nuts

3 tablespoons agave nectar, or to taste

¾–1 cup water or coconut water

½ teaspoon vanilla extract (optional)

1. Using your creative abilities, decorate a bowl with the banana slices and fresh berries.
2. Combine all the Crème de la Crème ingredients in a blender or food processor and blend until creamy. You will need to adjust the water depending upon the strength of your blender.
3. Top the fruit with a dollop of Crème de la Crème and garnish with the mint leaves.

Variations

- In addition to the berries, create the fruit salad of your dreams with peaches, nectarines, mangoes, papaya, and pineapple.
- Replace the macadamia nuts with cashews.
- For a supercreamy version of the Crème de la Crème, you can add ½ cup of medium-soft coconut meat (see page 29), or mashed banana.

> ### Quicker and Easier
>
> Açaí—the high antioxidant purple berry of the açaí palm, native to the Amazon, is most readily available in frozen form. For an energizing breakfast and popular way to enjoy this berry, blend some açaí with a banana or two, pour into a bowl, and top with your favorite granola.

MULTIGRAIN CEREAL

A step above a simple bowl of oatmeal, in this cereal the quinoa and kasha add a hint of nuttiness and create a grounding way to start the day, especially on cold winter mornings. Experimenting with the different grains and add-ons listed below will help you create a new hot cereal each day.

SERVES 2 TO 4

½ cup uncooked quinoa	Pinch of ground cinnamon
3¼ cups water	Pinch of ground cardamom
¼ cup uncooked kasha	Soy, rice, or nut milk (see page 42)
½ cup uncooked rolled oats	Pure maple syrup or agave nectar
1 medium-size banana, sliced	

1. Place the quinoa and water in a small pot over medium-low heat. Cook uncovered for 5 minutes.
2. Add the kasha and cook for 10 minutes, stirring occasionally.
3. Add the rolled oats, lower the heat to low, and cook, still uncovered, for about 7 minutes, or until all grains are cooked through, stirring frequently. Add additional water if necessary.
4. Add the banana, spices, and your nondairy milk of choice, and sweeten to taste.

Variations
- Try stirring 1 tablespoon of almond butter or other nut butter after cooking.
- Add your favorite fruits and dried fruits.
- You can add the banana with the oats while cooking, for an extra infusion of sweetness.
- Toast chopped walnuts or other nuts or seeds in a toaster oven for a few minutes at 350°F and add before serving.

If You Have More Time

Many variations are possible, using different grains. See the grain cooking chart on page 23 for cooking times. Consider rice and polenta as additions. Be daring and try a four-grain combination with your favorites.

TEMPEH BACON

If you love Babe, but still miss bacon, this recipe's for you. Below you'll find a healthier baked version and a more authentic fried version. Serve as part of a rocking brunch with Tofu Scramble (page 62) and Seasoned Spuds (page 68). If you want to go all out, add other accoutrements such as Pancakes (page 66) and French Toast (page 71).

SERVES 4

3 tablespoons soy sauce

3 tablespoons water

1 tablespoon pure maple syrup
or agave nectar

¼ teaspoon liquid smoke

½ teaspoon garlic powder

½ teaspoon onion powder

8 ounces tempeh,
sliced into thin strips

1. Place all the ingredients except the tempeh in a shallow dish and whisk well. Add the tempeh and marinate for 10 minutes, flipping frequently.
2. You have two options for cooking. A healthier version is to preheat the oven or a toaster oven to 350°F and place the tempeh on a well-oiled baking sheet. Bake for 8 minutes, flip, and bake for another 7 minutes.
3. For the full crispy, almost-like-bacon effect, place 2 tablespoons of coconut oil or your favorite oil in a medium-size sauté pan. Sauté the tempeh over medium-high heat until crispy, flipping occasionally to cook both sides evenly.

Variation
- You can replace the tempeh with 8 ounces of thinly sliced, extra-firm tofu. To create the slices, cut the block of tofu in half and then slice thinly.

Tips and Tricks

Try adding 1 teaspoon of smoked paprika (pimentón de la vera), if you can find it, instead of the liquid smoke in this recipe and others that call for liquid smoke. Smoked paprika can be ordered at the Spanish Table Web site, www.spanishtable.com.

COSMIC CREPES

Crepes are impressive, especially when folks learn after enjoying them thoroughly, that they are vegan. Although the crepe batter takes mere moments to whip up, making them involves patience, as each crepe can take up to four minutes to cook—but the extra effort is worth it! Crepes can be served solo, with a dab of butter and a sprinkle of brown sugar. However, these days, creperies are cranking out all kinds of variations. If you choose to make one of our fillings, understand that you'll have to work on them while your crepes are cooking up, to fit into the thirty-minute time frame. But both our sweet and savory filling recipes are so simple that you can easily do this, and you'll probably be happy to have something else to do during that time.

MAKES TEN 8-INCH CREPES

1½ cups unbleached all-purpose flour or white spelt flour (see Tips and Tricks)

½ teaspoon sea salt

1 tablespoon tapioca flour or arrowroot

2½ cups water

1 tablespoon safflower oil + extra for cooking

Vegan butter (optional)

Pure maple syrup or brown sugar (optional)

1. Heat your crepe or sauté pans over medium heat. Sift the flour, salt, and tapioca flour through a fine-mesh strainer or sifter into a large bowl. Whisk together. Add the water and oil, and whisk again until well combined.
2. If you are not using a nonstick pan, use only a very light coating of oil. Ideally, use a pastry brush to spread out a very small drop of oil. Use a ⅓-cup measuring cup to scoop the batter. Hold the pan at a 45-degree angle, pour in the batter at the top of the pan, and quickly swirl the pan in a circular motion to spread out the batter into a very thin layer. Adjust the amount of batter to suit the size of the pan you are using. The crepes should be very, very thin. Cook for about 3 minutes on the first side, or until bubbles appear over the whole crepe. Flip, and cook for about 1 more minute.
3. Fold the crepe in half, then in half again. Lay it on a plate or baking tray while you work on the others. Serve immediately with a generous helping of vegan butter and maple syrup or brown sugar. The ambitious cooks can serve with the fillings or toppings included on the following pages.

Tips and Tricks

Crepe pans look like large, flat sauté pans with shallow or no sides and a long handle. This is so that you can pick the pan up and swirl it around to make the batter into a thin, large circle. Understandably, you may not be interested in investing in one of these pans. Don't tell the French Culinary Institute that we said so, but you can have very good results using a regular sauté pan. Nonstick or very lightly oiled pans work quite well; cast-iron pans do not work so well. Since they take a while to cook up, we recommend using more than one pan at a time, even if they are different sizes.

Also, most crepe recipes you find are going to be made from all-purpose flour. This will provide the fluffiest crepe; however, since crepes are so flat, whole-grain flours also work well. Unlike pancakes, which are prized for their fluffiness, crepes are so thin that you can get away with a little more. Classically, savory crepes are made with buckwheat flour, sweet crepes are made with white wheat flour.

Variations

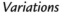

- If necessary, replace the tapioca flour with Egg Replacer from Ener-G Foods. Use the equivalent of one egg.
- Garbanzo bean flour makes good crepes as well. You can do a fifty-fifty mix with your favorite flour or try it with 100 percent garbanzo flour.
- Add flavor to your crepes by adding 1 teaspoon of orange zest or even lime zest. Also, play with extracts, such as vanilla, coffee, hazelnut, or even cherry—why not!

MUSHROOM-SPINACH CREPE FILLING

There's just something so delightful about the simplicity of mushrooms, garlic, olive oil, and salt. The addition of thin strips of spinach and basil takes it up a notch in both nutrition and flavor. This filling is one of our favorites!

MAKES 2½ CUPS

1 tablespoon olive oil

¾ pound cremini mushrooms,
thinly sliced (4 cups)

2 garlic cloves, pressed or minced

1 teaspoon soy sauce

¼ teaspoon sea salt

1 cup spinach, well washed,
sliced thinly, and tightly packed

½ cup fresh basil, cut in a chiffonade

1. Sauté the olive oil, mushrooms, garlic, soy sauce, and salt over medium heat for 5 minutes or until the mushrooms are tender, stirring frequently. You may wish to cover the pan for 1 to 2 minutes to bring out some of the juices of the mushrooms.
2. Transfer to a bowl, add the spinach and basil, and stir. Top or fill the crepes with your desired amount of filling.

STRAWBERRY-RHUBARB CREPE FILLING

This strawberry-rhubarb sauce is so absolutely pleasant. If you don't happen to hit that short window of frozen rhubarb availability, just add another cup of strawberries. Obviously, if you have access to fresh strawberries and/or rhubarb, this is by far the way to go. Just play with the quantities; you really can't mess it up.

MAKES ENOUGH FOR 10 CREPES

1 cup frozen strawberries, thawed

1 cup frozen rhubarb, thawed

¼ cup agave nectar

Pinch of sea salt

4 cups banana, cut into half-moons

1. Blend the strawberries, rhubarb, agave nectar, and salt until smooth.
2. Either fill the middle of a crepe with some sliced bananas and about 2 tablespoons of the sauce, or just top the crepes with both the bananas and the sauce and enjoy!

Variations

- This crepe filling would be even more lovely with ½ teaspoon of orange zest either added to the sauce or stirred in with the bananas and then covered in some lime juice.
- Some folks would agree that ¼ cup of grain-sweetened vegan dark chocolate chips would blend with the bananas quite well. Or use a grater to shave off some chocolate from your favorite bar.
- Top with some toasted and chopped macadamia nuts or almonds.

Quicker and Easier

No time to make crepes? Try using flour tortillas. One idea for a filling breakfast that is a snap to prepare is a tortilla with almond butter and banana. You can heat up the tortilla on a griddle or in a sauté pan, if you wish. You can slice the banana or leave it whole. This makes a quickie grab-and-go breakfast. Another idea is to try the crepe fillings with your hot tortilla!

TOFU SCRAMBLE

Nutritionally light years ahead of its egg counterpart, this scramble is one of our favorite recipes for introducing folks to tofu. Be sure to use extra-firm tofu. Watch as the turmeric creates a vibrant yellow in the dish. Serve with Seasoned Spuds (page 68) and Tempeh Bacon (page 57) for a hearty vegan breakfast.

SERVES 2 TO 4

1½ tablespoons safflower oil

1 cup yellow onion, chopped small

4 medium-size garlic cloves, pressed or minced

1 pound extra-firm tofu, crumbled into large chunks

¾ teaspoon powdered turmeric

¾ teaspoon paprika

3 tablespoons nutritional yeast

1½ teaspoons soy sauce, or to taste

Sea salt and black pepper

1. Place the oil in a large sauté pan over medium-high heat. Add the onion and garlic and cook until the onions are soft, about 3 minutes, stirring frequently.
2. Add the tofu. Cook for 5 minutes, stirring frequently.
3. Add the remaining ingredients, cook 3–5 minutes more, season to taste, and enjoy.

Variations

TOFU SCRAMBLE ITALIANO

SERVES 6

To the simple Tofu Scramble, add the following:

4 large mushrooms, sliced
1 medium-size tomato, chopped
1 small bunch spinach, rinsed and drained (about 3 cups)
1½ tablespoons minced fresh basil
1 teaspoon dried oregano

Follow the Tofu Scramble recipe. Add the mushrooms with the onions and garlic. Add the remaining ingredients at the end of step 3 before seasoning.

SOUTHWEST TOFU SCRAMBLE

SERVES 4

To the simple Tofu Scramble, add the following:

1 small red bell pepper, seeded and chopped
1 medium-size jalapeño or other chile pepper, seeded and minced
2 tablespoons minced fresh cilantro
1½ teaspoons chile powder
1 teaspoon ground cumin
½ cup salsa and/or corn kernels (optional)

Follow the Tofu Scramble recipe. Add the bell pepper and jalapeño with the onions and garlic. Add the remaining ingredients at the end of step 3 before seasoning.

ONION-ZUCCHINI CORN CAKES

For savory breakfast lovers, these little gems can really light up your morning repertoire. A little dollop of applesauce and/or Vegan Sour Cream (page 289) pushes it over the edge. We also "accidentally" discovered they are exceedingly resplendent with maple syrup.

MAKES EIGHT TO TEN 4-INCH CAKES

½ cup cornmeal

¼ cup whole spelt flour

½ teaspoon baking powder, sifted

½ teaspoon sea salt

2 tablespoons ground flaxseed

¼–½ cup rice milk

3 cups grated zucchini
(about 3 medium zucchinis)

1 medium-size yellow onion,
diced (about 1 cup)

½ cup green onion, sliced thinly

1 tablespoon minced fresh
Italian parsley

1. In a medium-size bowl, whisk the cornmeal, flour, baking powder, salt, flaxseeds, and ¼ cup of the rice milk. At this point you may want to preheat your griddle or skillet over low heat so that it is ready to go when the batter is finished.
2. Add the zucchini, onion, green onion, and parsley to the cornmeal mixture and stir well to make a chunky, hearty mixture. If necessary to achieve a thinner batter, add some or all of the remaining ¼ cup of rice milk (see Tips and Tricks).
3. Using a ⅓-cup measuring cup, scoop the mixture onto the hot skillet over low heat and use the bottom of the measuring cup to flatten them out so that they are not too thick. Thick cakes will not cook all the way through. Flip when the underside is browned. Remove from the pan when the second side is also browned. Serve immediately with your choice of condiments.

Tips and Tricks

As the corn cakes cook, the vegetables will release more of their liquid. Adding the entire additional ¼ cup of rice milk could result in moister corn cakes. You don't need much liquid, you want them to cook all the way through. Moister corn cakes are trickier to flip over. Alas, knowing just how much rice milk to add is a learning process so have fun with it; the results are always tasty.

Superfoods for Health

Flaxseeds are one of the original foods Hippocrates, the father of modern medicine, recommended when he said, "Let food be thy medicine, and thy medicine be food." Flax is a nutritional powerhouse, with many uses in the *30-Minute Vegan* kitchen. A plant-based source of protein and essential fatty acids, ground flax (or flax meal) is available at health food stores. You can also grind your own with a spice grinder or a strong blender. Often used as an egg replacer in vegan food preparation and baking, the ground flaxseeds create a binding effect in dishes.

"BUTTERMILK" PANCAKES

We employed the pickiest pancake eaters we could find (Erica and Neil Greene) to develop the most authentic "buttermilk" pancake recipe possible. Buttermilk is really just sour milk with a fancy name. Seasoned bakers make their own buttermilk and you can, too—without the milk! According to our pancake connoisseurs, the version made from the white wheat flour gets you those ultimately fluffy-licious flapjacks. Keep the heat low to ensure the middle cooks all the way through without the outsides getting too browned.

MAKES 10 TO 12 PANCAKES

1½ cups soy milk

1 tablespoon + 1 teaspoon freshly squeezed lemon juice or raw apple cider vinegar

2 cups whole or white spelt flour, or substitute unbleached all-purpose flour

1 tablespoon + 1 teaspoon baking powder, sifted

½ teaspoon ground cinnamon

¼ cup plain soy yogurt

1 tablespoon safflower or coconut oil

2 tablespoons pure maple syrup

Vegan butter or coconut oil, for cooking

1. To make the "buttermilk," pour the soy milk into a 2-cup measuring cup, add the lemon juice, stir gently, and allow it to sit out on the counter for 10 minutes.
2. Meanwhile, sift the flour, baking powder, and cinnamon into a mixing bowl and whisk together. At this point, start to heat up your skillet or griddle. You may want to oil it as well, using the vegan butter or coconut oil. Keep the heat on low.
3. Add the yogurt, safflower oil, and maple syrup to the buttermilk and whisk until well incorporated. Use a rubber spatula to combine the liquid with the flour mixture. Stir until just blended, do not overmix.
4. Pour ¼ cup of the batter onto the lightly oiled skillet over low heat. Do not try to spread the batter around. Just pour it on and it will spread out on its own. If it doesn't, you may need to add a little more soy milk to the batter (start with 2 tablespoons). Wait until the top is bubbly all the way through and then flip. The pancakes are ready when you see steam coming out from the bottom and the bottom looks light brown. Enjoy with your favorite toppings and homemade syrup (page 39).

Variations

- For blueberry, strawberry, or raspberry pancakes, add ¾ cup fresh berries as directed in the tip below.
- Add ½ cup vegan dark chocolate chips to entertain the child within you. (see tip below)
- Orange zest adds an uplifting effect. Start with 1 teaspoon. Lemon zest is nice as well, especially when you are adding blueberries. Or try orange raspberry.
- For banana-walnut pancakes, add ¾ cup of diced banana and ¼ cup of diced walnuts. You may also wish to add ¼ teaspoon of banana extract.
- Flavor up your flapjacks with any of your favorite extracts and flavors such as vanilla, orange, or almond. Or be daring with hazelnut, coconut, or coffee!

Tips and Tricks

When adding ingredients to pancakes, such as fruit and chocolate chips, it is advisable to leave these out of the actual batter and keep them in a bowl next to you while you are cooking. Pour the pancakes onto the griddle or pan and then sprinkle with your desired accoutrements. This is the best way to keep the pancakes from sticking and the fillings from burning. Flavorings, zest, and extracts should be stirred into the batter directly before pouring.

SEASONED SPUDS

No matter how many diets come and go that try to oust the potato from the culinary spotlight, the spuds just don't budge. Here we offer a fresher version of the classic roasted potato. The unheated oil is a much healthier way to go and it is amazing how much less time potatoes take to steam compared to roasting or boiling. Serve with virtually all of the breakfast and brunch recipes or on their own with a side of Vegan Sour Cream (page 289).

SERVES 4 TO 6

4 medium-size russet potatoes, cut into ½-inch cubes (about 5½ cups)

1 teaspoon fennel seeds

2 tablespoons olive oil

1 tablespoon minced fresh rosemary

2 garlic cloves, pressed or minced

2 teaspoons soy sauce

1 teaspoon paprika

½ teaspoon black pepper

¼ teaspoon sea salt, or to taste

1. Start the water boiling in your steamer while you are chopping the potatoes. Steam the potatoes until you can easily pass a fork through the ones on the top, 10 to 15 minutes (red, purple, or other potatoes may take longer).
2. Meanwhile, heat the fennel seeds in a sauté pan over medium-high heat until they smell toasty, about 2 minutes. Transfer to a mixing bowl and add the olive oil, rosemary, garlic, soy sauce, paprika, pepper, and salt. Stir well. Add the steamed potatoes and stir gently. Serve hot.

Variations

- You'll love the Mexican version of this recipe. Omit the fennel seeds and rosemary, and substitute 1 teaspoon of chile powder, 1 teaspoon of ground cumin, and ½ teaspoon of cayenne. Serve with a side of Salsa (page 82) and Vegan Sour Cream (page 289), and top with copious amounts of minced fresh cilantro.
- You can also use your favorite dried and fresh herbs, such as thyme, parsley, marjoram, or oregano.

♥
LIVE CINNAMON ROLLS

These puppies are a huge hit at our bakery in Kaua'i. The rolling technique is best carried out with the use of a Silpat (silicon baking sheet), Teflex sheet (used in dehydrators), or a baking sheet lined with parchment paper. You'll also need a food processor. The icing is not necessary for you to enjoy this dish but pushes it into the decadent category. Cashews can be substituted for the coconut butter in the icing if you cannot find it or you don't have a taste for coconut.

MAKES 12 ROLLS

2 cups raw buckwheat groats
(not kasha)

2 cups + ½ cup pitted
Medjool dates, packed

2 tablespoons + 1 teaspoon agave nectar

¼ cup water

2 tablespoons ground cinnamon

Pinch of sea salt

¼ cup raisins

½ cup walnuts, chopped

Icing (optional)

½ cup coconut butter
(not coconut oil)

¼ cup agave nectar

½ teaspoon vanilla extract

1 tablespoon orange zest

¼ cup water or freshly squeezed
orange juice

1. Process the buckwheat groats for 60 seconds in a food processor, or until they are finely ground. There will still be some whole kernels. Add 2 cups of the dates and continue to process for about 40 seconds. Add 1 teaspoon of the agave nectar and process for 30 seconds more, or until a sticky "dough" forms. If a piece of dough can be formed into a tight little ball, it is ready, otherwise add 1 teaspoon at a time of agave nectar until this desired stickiness is reached.

2. Transfer the dough to a flat work surface covered with a Silpat, a Teflex sheet, or parchment paper. Using your hands, press the dough into a rectangle that is roughly 9 x 11 inches and ¼ inch thick. Keep some water nearby to dip your fingers into, to prevent the dough from sticking to them. Position the dough so that the long side is parallel with the counter's edge.

3. Process the remaining ½ cup of dates, 2 tablespoons of agave nectar, water, cinnamon, and salt in the food processor until as smooth as possible. There will probably be chunks because the quantity of mixture may be too small to process thoroughly. Remove the processor blade and stir in the raisins and walnuts. Spread the mixture over all of the dough except for about 1 inch along the far long edge.

4. Roll up the dough by making a small fold along the near long edge, pressing it down, peeling back the Silpat, and continuing to roll in the same way, making sure to press the whole thing together as you go so that you have a tight roll. Refrigerate while you make the icing and then cut the log into twelve even slices.
5. Blend all of the icing ingredients until smooth. Either drizzle it over the whole log or over the individual slices. There should be more than enough icing.

Variations

- For a more devilish dessert, try making a Chocolate-Mint Roll by adding ½ cup raw cacao powder to the dough in step 1. Omit the cinnamon, add ¼ cup of raw cacao powder, and ½ teaspoon of peppermint extract to the filling in step 3. Also, in step 3 you can add 2 tablespoons of raw cacao nibs along with the raisins, and replace the walnuts with macadamia nuts or omit them altogether.
- Another richer variation would be to replace the buckwheat groats with an equal amount of almonds. Simply make almond flour in a high-powered blender or food processor and continue with the recipe.

Superfoods for Health

With origins in Ancient China and popular in Eastern Europe, buckwheat is a triangular-shaped fruit seed often considered a grain. It's not related to wheat and is entirely gluten free. Raw groats are used in live food preparation. The roasted groat is kasha. Among other nutritional qualities, buckwheat is high in rutin, a bioflavonoid with antioxidant properties that is vital for blood vessel health.

MAPLE-ALMOND FRENCH TOAST

Mark has pleasant memories of eating challah French toast almost every Saturday morning, while growing up. For those not wishing to go through the trouble of making a vegan challah, buy an unsliced loaf of bread and cut thick slices. We love ours served with almond butter, flaxseed oil, and maple syrup or homemade syrup (page 39). Another favorite way to enjoy this is to sprinkle with cinnamon and top with fresh fruit (try mango—yum!).

MAKES 10 SLICES (LESS IF USING THICKER SLICES)

1 recipe French Toast Batter
(see below)

Vegan butter or oil of choice

10 slices bread of choice

French Toast Batter

1¼ cups soy, rice, or coconut milk,
or soy creamer

½ teaspoon ground cinnamon

¼ teaspoon ground allspice

2 tablespoons almond butter or
tahini or a combination of both

3 tablespoons flour
(try spelt or buckwheat)

½ teaspoon vanilla extract

1 tablespoon pure maple syrup,
Sucanat, organic sugar,
or sweetener of choice

1 tablespoon ground flaxseeds
(optional)

1. Preheat a griddle or large cast-iron pan over medium-high heat. Combine the batter ingredients in a large bowl and whisk well.
2. Place a small amount of vegan butter on the griddle. Dip the bread slices into the batter, coating both sides well, and place on the griddle. (Three or four slices should fit simultaneously on a griddle or large cast-iron pan.) Flip after a few minutes, to prevent sticking.
3. Cook until browned on both sides, about 5 minutes, adding more vegan butter to the griddle if necessary to avoid sticking. Rewhisk the remaining batter between dipping the bread slices. Serve the toast with toppings of choice.

Quicker and Easier

As an alternative to buttered toast, try whole-grain bread, toast, or rice crackers with flax or hemp oil, almond butter, and jam. For a savory start, top with vegan butter or your favorite oil, nutritional yeast, and a pinch of salt. Be adventurous and add a bit of miso paste, tomato, avocado, red onion, and cucumber.

COCONUT-LIME BANANA BREAD

If you count baking time, this recipe does exceed the thirty-minute time frame. The preparation, however, will only take about twenty minutes. We included it because this bread beats the pants off plain ol' banana bread. If you have the time, you should definitely take the extra few minutes to make the ultra-epic glaze topping. If you choose not to use coconut oil, you could add 1 teaspoon of coconut extract along with the vanilla. The recipe suggests using a standing mixer but you could also use a hand mixer or mix by hand if necessary. A food processor also works for mixing the wet ingredients but avoid blending, which may add too much air to the mixture. Lastly, a good zester is key, but decent results can be achieved with the fine side of a cheese grater.

MAKES 1 STANDARD LOAF OR 3 MINI LOAVES

2 cups whole spelt flour

1 teaspoon baking soda

½ teaspoon sea salt

½ cup shredded coconut

1½ cups banana, sliced
(or mashed if preparing by hand)

½ cup coconut, safflower,
or sunflower oil

1 cup Sucanat

1 tablespoon vanilla extract or
Jamaican Rum

¼ cup soy yogurt

1 teaspoon raw apple cider vinegar

1 teaspoon lime zest

Glaze

¼ cup agave nectar

1 tablespoon freshly squeezed
lime juice

1 teaspoon lime zest

½ cup shredded coconut
(optional)

1. Preheat the oven to 350°F. Lightly oil the baking pans and dust with flour. Sift the spelt flour, baking soda, and salt through a fine-mesh strainer. Add the shredded coconut, whisk it all together, and set aside.
2. In the bowl of a standing mixer with the paddle attachment, start to blend the banana on low speed, changing to medium speed as the banana mashes more. Add the oil, Sucanat, vanilla, yogurt, vinegar, and zest, and keep blending for 2 minutes, or until the mixture is uniform and soupy with very few chunks of banana.
3. Reduce the speed to low and slowly add the flour mixture. If using a hand mixer, stir in flour by hand. Blend for 1 minute, or until the dough is blended but still chunky. Do not overmix! It doesn't need to look like pancake batter; chunks are okay. Transfer to the prepared baking pan(s).

4. Bake for 60 minutes for a standard loaf pan or 40 minutes for the mini loaves, or until a toothpick in the center comes out clean and the edges have pulled away from the pan. Remove from the oven and let the pan sit for 10 to 15 minutes before removing the bread and transferring it to a wire rack.
5. For the glaze, combine all of the ingredients together and let it sit while the bread bakes. Pour it over the bread after it is transferred from the pan to the wire rack. Try to keep most of the coconut, if using, on the top. It will stick more as the bread continues to cool.

Some folks insist on letting banana bread sit overnight because its flavor and texture enhance with time. Others cannot wait to tear into it while it is still warm from the oven. Either way, you really can't lose. But be forewarned that the aroma of this bread in the oven stirs the appetite immensely.

Variations
- Add ½ cup of your favorite nuts, such as walnuts, macadamia nuts, or toasted almonds.
- Experiment with different flavors and extracts, such as almond, orange, and lemon.
- Use orange juice and orange zest where the lime is called for.
- Try toasting the shredded coconut for the bread and/or the topping (see page 26).

BREAKFAST BURRITO

This is the ultimate solution to leftover Tofu Scramble (see page 62). You want to use the largest whole-grain flour tortillas possible for the burrito grande. Experiment with different beans and/or other tofu dishes as the filling (see suggestions below). For best results, and if you have the time, serve with Guacamole (page 88), Salsa (page 82), and Vegan Sour Cream (page 289).

SERVES 4 TO 6

1 (15-ounce) can black beans, or 1½ cups cooked

1 teaspoon chile powder

1 teaspoon ground cumin

2 garlic cloves, pressed or minced (optional)

1 small jalapeño, seeded and minced (optional)

Sea salt

1 recipe Tofu Scramble (page 62)

2 to 3 small tomatoes

¼ cup minced fresh cilantro

4 to 6 large tortillas

1. Place the beans and the liquid from the can or a little water in a small pot over low heat. Add the chile powder, cumin, garlic, and jalapeño, if using. Cook for 10 minutes, stirring occasionally. Add salt to taste.
2. While the beans are cooking, prepare the Tofu Scramble. Chop the tomatoes and mince the cilantro. Heat a tortilla on a skillet or in a pan until warm.
3. Place about ½ cup of the Tofu Scramble, ¼ cup of beans, and your desired amount of tomato and cilantro in the center of the tortilla. Fold in the sides and roll away from you. For a nice presentation, slice in half diagonally before serving.

Variations
- Replace the Tofu Scramble with another tofu dish, such as Tofu Satay (page 193) or Tofu-Garden Vegetable Salad (page 148).
- Try with pinto, kidney, or your favorite beans.

If You Have More Time
Replace the tomatoes with Salsa (page 82) and add some Vegan Sour Cream (page 289) and Hot Sauce (page 281). The Seasoned Spuds (page 68) make another delish filling for this burrito.

CHILAQUILES

One of the ways the women of Mexico devised to make use of stale tortillas, which they had belabored themselves to make by hand, is Chilaquiles. This dish is served in practically as many ways as there are families in Mexico but generally consists of the tortilla strips swimming in a sea of red or green sauce (a soupy sort of salsa) perhaps with a bit of meat or scrambled eggs and topped with queso blanco (a mild white cheese). Chilaquiles are also a renowned hangover cure for those in the know.

SERVES 4

Salsa
8 medium Roma tomatoes
½ red bell pepper, seeded
½ green bell pepper, seeded
½ yellow onion, layers separated
4 garlic cloves
¼ cup chopped fresh cilantro
1 teaspoon soy sauce
½ teaspoon sea salt
½ teaspoon black pepper
1 tablespoon freshly squeezed lime juice
¼ teaspoon celery seeds

To sauté and assemble
1 tablespoon olive oil
½ yellow onion, chopped
½ red bell pepper, seeded and sliced
½ green bell pepper, seeded and sliced
1 garlic clove, pressed or minced
1 (8-ounce) package seitan, separated into small pieces
4 ounces tortilla chips, stale or fresh
½ cup grated vegan mozzarella
¼ cup minced fresh cilantro

1. Set the broiler to high. Cut a cone-shaped hole into the top of the tomatoes, using a paring knife, removing most of the core. Arrange the tomatoes (top

continues

side down), bell pepper halves, onion, and garlic on a baking tray with sides or a casserole dish. Broil for 15 minutes and remove from the oven. You may wish to flip them with tongs halfway through, to ensure even cooking.

2. Remove the garlic bulbs from their skins, and transfer them along with the other broiled veggies, and the remaining salsa ingredients to the blender or food processor, and blend at high speed until smooth.

3. While the vegetables are broiling, sauté the olive oil, onion, bell peppers, garlic, and seitan in a sauté pan over medium heat for 8 to 10 minutes, until the vegetables are tender, stirring frequently.

4. To serve, arrange the sautéed vegetables on a plate, top with a handful of tortillas, cover with the salsa, and top with the mozzarella and cilantro.

Tips and Tricks

Unlike tofu and tempeh, which are made from soy, seitan is made from wheat gluten. It is high in protein and can be used in recipes the same way animal products would be used, with little or no adjustments to the recipe. Seitan may be stored in the refrigerator for about one week when out of its packaging or it may be frozen for longer-term storage.

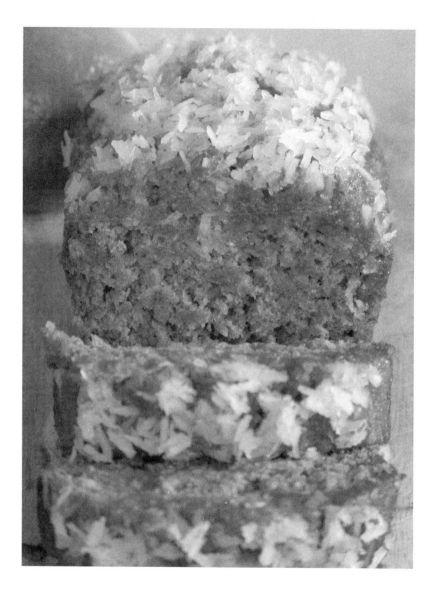

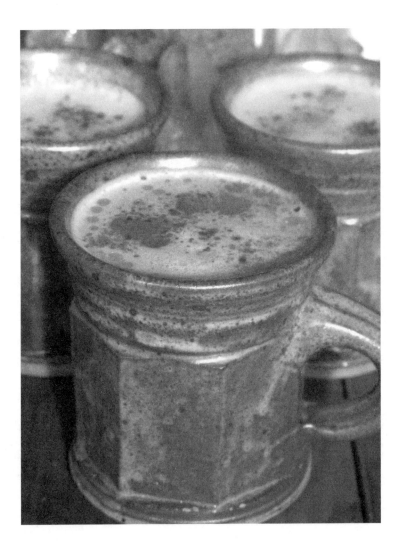

CHAPTER 5

Snacks, Pick-Me-Ups, and Kids' Favorites

One question we get asked frequently is, "What do you eat every day?" Often we hear this at one of our cooking classes, after we had just spent hours talking about the many possible variations of the food we were demonstrating. Baffled by this time and time again, we finally started asking folks to clarify the question. It turns out that what most people want to know is what kinds of things we whip up when we aren't in the mood to make a big hullabaloo. Or even a little kerfuffle.

The funny thing is, as people in the business of making food can relate to, we usually make only the simplest foods at home. We aren't out to impress each other at all and we are both easily satisfied. This chapter highlights those quick and easy between-meals type foods that we throw together whenever the mood strikes us. A quick, fresh salsa to go with some chips or crackers, mochi pizza, corn on the cob, and rich, satisfying hot chocolate are the kinds of goodies that tie us over until something a little more substantial comes along.

POPSICLES

Everyone loves a cold sweet treat on a blazing hot day. Or the night after a blazing hot day. Or a breezy day when the sun hits the porch just right. Heck, any ol' time is a good time for a Popsicle. Here are three tantalizing options in the endless world of Popsicle creation. With all of the exotic jarred juices and juice blends, the sky's the limit. While they do require freezing for a few hours, preparing them is as simple as turning on a blender.

MAKES 4 TO 8 POPS

Antioxicles

½ heaping cup blueberries

½ heaping cup raspberries

1 cup pomegranate juice

1 tablespoon agave nectar, optional

Tropsicles

1 cup pineapple, chopped

1 cup coconut nectar, or coconut-based beverage
(available in most health food stores; Knudsen offers a good product)

1 medium-size banana

¼ teaspoon vanilla extract

1 tablespoon agave nectar (optional)

Fudgsicles

1½ cups chocolate soy milk

¼ cup almond butter

2 tablespoons unsweetened
cocoa powder

½ teaspoon vanilla extract

3 tablespoons pure maple syrup

1. Blend all of the ingredients together, pour into a Popsicle tray and insert the sticks, and freeze for at least a few hours on a flat space in the freezer.
2. Once solid, defrost for 5 minutes, or you may wish to rinse the tray under running water to loosen the pops. Otherwise you'll end up with a stick in your hand and the Popsicle still in the tray. Enjoy!

HOT CHOCOLATE

We vigorously debated which chapter to place this recipe in. While certainly a beverage, it is also a popular comfort food. We broke the deadlock by placing it in the kids' favorites chapter. This version uses natural sweeteners rather than the refined sugars found in commercial hot chocolate mixes. Use soy milk for the creamiest version. The raw variation is a superfood tonic that will leave you energized for hours.

MAKES TWO 10-OUNCE SERVINGS

2½ cups soy or rice milk

¼ cup unsweetened cocoa powder

2–3 tablespoons pure maple syrup or agave nectar, or to taste

1. Heat the soy milk in a small pot on low heat for a few minutes; do not allow it to boil.
2. Whisk in the cocoa powder and maple syrup to taste. For a luscious addition, consider melting in vegan dark chocolate.

Variation

- ♥ **Raw Incan Chocolate Tonic**: Replace the soy milk with almond, Brazil, or macadamia nut milk (see page 42); replace the cocoa powder with raw cacao powder; add ½ teaspoon of maca powder and the seeds from ½ vanilla bean (optional); and use agave nectar to taste, instead of the maple syrup. Place in a blender and blend until creamy. Enjoy cold, or heat it on the stove until warm to the touch.

Superfoods for Health

Cacao is the nutrient-rich, antioxidant power food of the Aztecs, Incans, and Mayans. Its scientific name, *Theobroma*, translates as "food of the gods." Who would have thought? It's readily available as nibs, which are small bits of the cacao bean. It is also available in powdered form, both raw and roasted. Maca root is a Peruvian tuber, purported to improve vitality and mental clarity. It is commonly available in powdered form in most health food stores. The combination of these two superfoods creates a synergistic burst of energy.

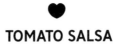

TOMATO SALSA

Use this recipe to create every type of salsa imaginable (see Variations). If you have time, let the salsa sit for twenty minutes before serving, for the flavors to deepen. Taking the time to toast the spices beforehand also enhances the flavor. Serve with chips for a quick snack and to complement all of your Mexican fiestas.

MAKES 2½ CUPS

2 large tomatoes, chopped
¼ cup diced red onion
2 tablespoons minced fresh cilantro
2 tablespoons freshly squeezed lime juice
½ teaspoon minced garlic
1 teaspoon seeded and minced jalapeño (optional)
½ teaspoon chile powder
¼ teaspoon ground cumin
Pinch of cayenne
Sea salt and black pepper

Place all of the ingredients in a large mixing bowl and mix well.

Variations
- Try toasting the cumin and chile powder (see page 26).
- For a new kick, replace the tomatoes with papaya, mangoes, pineapple, or tomatillos.
- For a heartier flavor, add ¼ cup toasted pine nuts or toasted pumpkin seeds (see page 90).
- Add 1 cup cooked and cooled (or one 15-ounce can of drained and rinsed) black beans for a more substantial salsa.

Flavored Popcorn

In our circle of friends, there is a profound love and respect for popcorn. We like to invent fun and exciting flavors. Here are three of our favorites. Some like it hot, some like it sweet, and some like it green! All are a lot of fun at parties. Frequently the spirulina variety sits around getting a lot of sideways glances until some adventurous child decides to give the weird stuff a whirl. Next thing you know, it's the talk of the town. Discerning popcorn aficionados covet the white variety of popcorn, which yields smaller, whiter popcorn that is considerably crisper and crunchier than the yellow kind.

HOT & SPICY POPCORN

SERVES 2 TO 4

½ cup popcorn kernels

1 tablespoon olive oil

1 tablespoon nutritional yeast

½ teaspoon chile powder

¼ teaspoon garlic powder

¼ teaspoon cayenne

¼ teaspoon sea salt, or to taste

1. Pop the corn in an air popper or by the method described in Tips and Tricks. Transfer the popped corn to a clean brown paper bag.
2. Drizzle the olive oil as evenly as possible over the top while shaking it up a little bit. Then add the nutritional yeast, chile powder, garlic powder, cayenne, and salt.
3. Close the top of the bag and shake vigorously. Pour into a bowl and enjoy!

KISS ME AT THE MOVIES CINNAMON-SUGAR POPCORN

SERVES 2 TO 4

½ cup popcorn kernels

1 tablespoon coconut oil

1 tablespoon Sucanat, turbinado sugar, or organic sugar

¾ teaspoon ground cinnamon

Pinch of sea salt

1. Pop the corn in an air popper or by the method described in Tips and Tricks. Transfer the popped corn to a clean brown paper bag.
2. Drizzle the coconut oil as evenly as possible over the top while shaking it up a little bit. Then add the Sucanat, cinnamon, and salt.
3. Close the top of the bag and shake vigorously. Pour into a bowl and enjoy!

SPIRULINA POPCORN

SERVES 2 TO 4

½ cup popcorn kernels

1 tablespoon olive oil

2 tablespoons nutritional yeast

1 tablespoon spirulina

¼ teaspoon sea salt, or to taste

1. Pop the corn in an air popper or by the method described in Tips and Tricks. Transfer the popped corn to a clean brown paper bag.
2. Drizzle the olive oil as evenly as possible over the top while shaking it up a little bit. Then add the nutritional yeast, spirulina, and salt.
3. Close the top of the bag and shake vigorously. Pour into a bowl and get ready to open some minds to the joy of spirulina!

Tips and Tricks

The way you choose to pop your corn is up to you. Either you have a handy-dandy air popper, in which case you just add the popcorn, plug in the machine, and wait for fluffy popcorn. Otherwise you do it the old-fashioned way, which actually yields crunchier, fluffier popcorn. In this case, cover the bottom of a heavy-bottomed pot (make sure it has a lid!) with 2 to 4 tablespoons of safflower or co-conut oil. The trick to the crunchiness is not putting the popcorn in until the oil is hot enough to pop it. So throw in two or three kernels, cover with the lid, and wait until they all pop. Then quickly open the lid, toss the rest in, and replace the cover. The popcorn should start popping like crazy within a minute. Shake vigorously to avoid burning. Transfer to a brown paper bag or bowl immediately when you hear the pops minimize to one every few seconds.

Superfoods for Health

Jennifer's double-top-secret spirulina popcorn recipe is one of the tastiest ways to enjoy the superfood spirulina. Spirulina is a freshwater, blue-green algae containing protein, fatty acids, most B vitamins, as well as vitamins C, D, and E. Try it in smoothies, live pie fillings and crusts, or sprinkled on salads.

CRISPY KALE

Sure, sure, your kids don't like kale. But they haven't ever tried Crispy Kale, now have they? This recipe, ingeniously developed by our sister-in-law, Elizabeth, is the reason why we can't keep kale in the house. Scrumptious, nutritious, and crispy make a winning combination for all ages. Some people like it really crispy, some prefer a little chewiness—play with the baking time to see which you prefer. This recipe works best with curly-leaf kale. The flat kinds just don't crisp up the same.

SERVES 4 TO 6

1 large bunch curly-leaf kale
2 tablespoons olive oil
3 tablespoons nutritional yeast
½ teaspoon sea salt

1. Preheat the oven (or even a toaster oven for smaller batches) to 350°F. Use your hands to rip small pieces of the leaves off the stem of the kale. Arrange them on a baking sheet in a single layer, using two baking sheets if necessary. When the oven is ready, bake for 12 to 15 minutes, or until your desired crispiness is achieved.
2. Remove from the oven and transfer the kale to a large mixing bowl. Drizzle with the olive oil, sprinkle with the nutritional yeast and sea salt, and toss gently with your hands until all the kale is covered. Serve immediately, or store in an airtight container at room temperature. Please do not refrigerate.

Quicker and Easier

Almost everyone loves corn on the cob, especially during summer months when corn is abundant. A common way to prepare one of America's all-time favorites is to place the cobs in boiling water for a few minutes. Remove (tongs come in handy here) and enjoy with one of the variations below. You can also grill the cobs, being sure to baste often with oil or BBQ Sauce (page 123). Many enjoy corn raw on the cob. If you haven't tried it raw, you might be pleasantly surprised.

Here are three ways amongst many to partake:

- Slather in vegan butter and top with nutritional yeast, salt, and pepper to taste.
- Squeeze fresh lime juice on top, drizzle with olive oil, sprinkle with a pinch of chile powder, salt, and cayenne to taste.
- Go Italiano with a splash of balsamic vinegar, olive oil, minced fresh basil and parsley, sea salt, and freshly ground black pepper.

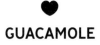

GUACAMOLE

What quick and easy vegan cookbook would be complete without a guacamole? Keep the seed in the dish to preserve the color and to make an intriguing conversation piece at parties. Serve as a snack with chips, a spread in any number of wraps (page 105), or use as part of our Breakfast Burrito (page 74).

MAKES 1½ CUPS

3 small avocados, seeded and chopped (1½ cups)

3 tablespoons diced red onion

1 tablespoon freshly squeezed lime juice

2 tablespoons minced fresh cilantro

1½ teaspoons seeded and minced
jalapeño pepper

1 teaspoon minced garlic

¼ teaspoon chile powder

Pinch of cayenne

Sea salt and black pepper

Place all of the ingredients in a mixing bowl and mix well, making sure to mash up the avocado well with a fork, yet leaving some chunks.

Variations

- Add ½ teaspoon of toasted ground cumin (see page 26).
- Add 1 tablespoon of Vegan Sour Cream (page 289).
- Add ¼ cup of Salsa (page 82) or diced tomatoes.
- For a distinctly robust guacamole, try increasing the quantity of red onion to ¼ cup, and double the amounts of cilantro, garlic, jalapeño, and lime juice. If you can get to a Mexican market, experiment with different flavored chile powders; smoky chipotle is our favorite.

Quicker and Easier

Simple Avocado Dip: Scoop out avocado, mash with a fork, and add salt to taste. Add ½ teaspoon of your favorite spice, such as curry powder, chile powder, or ground cumin. Use as a dip for cucumbers, carrots, crackers, or tortilla chips.

Superfoods for Health

Avocados, also called alligator pears because of their skin, are an ancient fruit that has been traced back to archaeological sites in Peru as far back as the eighth century BC. With almost one thousand different varieties, Hass is a popular choice. A source of beneficial fatty acids, avocados are said to be good for heart health when enjoyed in moderation. You can ripen them by placing in a paper bag or in a basket with other fruits. A ripe avocado is slightly soft to the touch. To check for ripeness you can also remove the stem and insert a toothpick. If the toothpick goes in easily, it is ready to eat or refrigerate. Do not refrigerate an unripe avocado.

SAVORY TOASTED PEPITAS

Toasted pumpkin seeds, or pepitas, are a fabulous snack for the trail or the beach, or to hold you over at work until your next meal. They are functional, easy to carry around with you, and have that addictive crunch power. We jazzed them up a little for your enjoyment.

MAKES 1 CUP

1 cup hulled pumpkin seeds
1 tablespoon soy sauce
1 teaspoon pure maple syrup
1 teaspoon toasted sesame oil
1 teaspoon umeboshi plum vinegar or raw apple cider vinegar

1. Preheat an oven or toaster oven to 350°F. Place the pumpkin seeds on a baking tray and toast for about 4 minutes, or until they just start to brown.
2. Meanwhile, mix together the soy sauce, maple syrup, toasted sesame oil, and vinegar. Toss the seeds with the mixture, and put them back in the oven for about 10 minutes, stirring once or twice. Don't worry if they are still a little wet; they will dry out as they cool.
3. Let them cool for about 5 minutes before breaking them apart with your hands.

Variations
- Try the same recipe with sunflower seeds or your favorite nuts.

Quicker and Easier

We actually love snacking on plain toasted pepitas on their own as a crunchy snack. You can toast them for a few minutes in a sauté pan over medium heat. They are done when they puff up and start to brown.

Trail Mixes

The fun thing about making your own trail mixes is not having to pick through to find the things that you like. You like everything! So mix it up—use your favorite nuts, seeds, dried fruits, even candies. These three recipes are but a few possibilities among thousands.

THE TEX-MEX MIX

Glad corn is a regular field corn that is "exploded," using heat. The result is quite like those half-popped kernels at the bottom of the popcorn bowl, only larger and more satisfying with much less chance of chipping a tooth. We love it alone as well as in this blend where it brings a taste of the Wild (Mid) West to your fingertips.

MAKES 2½ CUPS

1 cup glad corn
(or substitute mini pretzels)
½ cup almonds
½ cup cashews
½ cup peanuts
½ teaspoon chile powder
½ teaspoon garlic powder
½ teaspoon cayenne
¼ teaspoon liquid smoke
¼ teaspoon sea salt
2 teaspoons nutritional yeast

1. Mix all of the ingredients together and stir well.
2. Store in an airtight container for up to a week.

LEAVE NO TRAIL MIX

This is an example of a simplified trail mix that omits all those pesky ingredients that get left at the bottom of the bag. Leave out the carob chips for a ♥ live version.

MAKES 3 CUPS

¾ cup dried pineapple, chopped small

½ cup dried cranberries

1 cup walnuts

1 cup almonds

½ cup carob chips (optional)

1. Mix up all of the ingredients.
2. If you're including the carob chips, you may want to keep this refrigerated until you're ready to eat it or take it on the go.

Quicker and Easier

For a quick and nutritious snack, try boiled edamame with some sea salt or soy sauce. Edamame are soybeans that are harvested before they get too hard. Translated as "beans on branches," they grow in clusters on bushy branches. Usually found in the frozen section (both in the shell and shelled) edamame are parboiled before packaging. Simply place in boiling water for a few minutes, drain, and enjoy.

IS THERE ANY MORE OF THAT CHOCOLATE TRAIL MIX

This trail mix leaves all the others in the shadows. People can't keep their hands off it. The toastiness of the nuts, the sweetness of the chocolate, and the chewiness of the raisins are a winning combination. Try sprinkling it over sweet crepes, pancakes, waffles, or pudding. Be sure to wait until the nuts have cooled before mixing them in with the chocolate or you will melt the chips and have a mound of mix on your hands. There are worse problems really but. . . .

MAKES 2½ CUPS

1 cup pecans

1 cup macadamia nuts

¼ cup grain-sweetened dark chocolate chips

¼ cup raisins or currants

Pinch of sea salt

1. Chop and toast the nuts. You may wish to use a food processor to coarsely chop the pecans and macadamia nuts, and toast according to instructions on page 90.
2. After the pecans and macadamia nuts have thoroughly cooled, mix them together with the chocolate chips, raisins, and salt. Stir 'em up and enjoy.

Quicker and Easier

One of the best quick and easy snacks is apple slices, celery sticks, or banana slices with almond butter or your favorite nut butter. Adventurous souls can also sprinkle on a little cinnamon.

POWER-PACKED ENERGY BAR

Energy bars are big business these days. There are countless varieties on the market, each touting different claims. Here is a down-home version, courtesy of Jessyka Murray (Jennifer's sister), which is sure to provide a burst of energy.

MAKES 12 BARS

1 cup almonds

1 cup pecans or macadamia nuts

1 cup sunflower seeds

1 cup dried cranberries

½ cup dried shredded coconut

1 cup agave nectar

1 tablespoon coconut oil

1 tablespoon carob powder

1 teaspoon vanilla extract

½ teaspoon sea salt

1. Preheat the oven to 350°F and oil a 9 x 13-inch baking pan well. Grind the nuts into small pieces, using a food processor. Transfer to a mixing bowl with the seeds, dried fruit, and shredded coconut, and mix together.
2. Combine the agave, coconut oil, carob powder, vanilla, and salt in a small mixing bowl, and whisk until all of the lumps disappear. Pour the wet ingredients into the nut mixture and stir together with a rubber spatula until all is well coated.
3. Press into the prepared baking pan and bake for 15 minutes. Allow to cool for 10 minutes before cutting into twelve bars.

If You Have More Time

♥ For a live version, replace the agave nectar with 2 cups of pitted dates and reduce the sunflower seeds and cranberries to ½ cup each. Process the dates along with the nuts at the beginning of the recipe. Follow the rest of the recipe above except instead of baking, form twelve individual bars, place on a baking pan, and refrigerate for 30 minutes or longer.

For the ultimate energy bar, add 1 tablespoon of spirulina powder, 1 teaspoon of maca powder, and ¼ cup cacao nibs in with the dry ingredients and proceed with the recipe.

GRILLED PEANUT BUTTER AND JELLY

Who needs another peanut butter and jelly recipe? You will be pleasantly surprised how grilling transports this old favorite to the next level of tasty goodness! The secret to an epic Grilled PB&J is in the slow cooking which allows time for the middle to heat up. The way the warm peanut butter melts in your mouth next to the gooey fruit jelly is an unparalleled culinary achievement. Along with the crispy, buttery bread, you may find yourself heating up the skillet with great frequency. We highly recommend strawberry jam and crunchy peanut butter but we know we're stepping on some toes here.

SERVES 2

4 pieces bread of choice
Peanut butter
Sugar-free fruit preserves
Vegan butter or oil

1. Assemble the sandwich with your desired amount of fillings. We highly recommend generous quantities. Spread the vegan butter lightly on the outside of the bread.
2. In a skillet over medium-low heat, slowly brown both sides of the bread. Keep the heat rather low or the filling won't get hot and gooey enough before the bread toasts.

Variations

- Feel free to add your favorite fruits, nuts, seeds, and so on to the filling. Some of our favorites are: sliced bananas, chopped walnuts, cacao nibs, or chocolate chips—all great ways to have fun with this lunchtime classic!

PITA TRIANGLE TEA SANDWICHES

Kids love this super simple snack to satisfy between-meal hunger. Pita bread has a tendency to harden as it cools. For best results, enjoy while still warm.

MAKES 8 TRIANGLES

2 pitas

½ cup vegan cream cheese, or to taste

1 tomato, sliced into 8 thin slices

8 slices cucumber

¼ cup nutritional yeast

Sea salt

1. Warm the pitas in a skillet. Spread each pita with 2 tablespoons of the cream cheese.
2. Slice into quarters, top with tomato and cucumber slices, and sprinkle with nutritional yeast and salt.

Variations
- We listed the easiest version in the recipe. You can replace the cream cheese with Hummus (page 108), Garlic-Herb Aioli (page 290), or Macadamia Ricotta (page 219).
- Grown-ups may like to add red onion slices, arugula, and sliced olives.

ENGLISH MUFFIN MELTS

Once the fare of the Victorian England servant class, where they are called crumpets, the humble English muffin is now a favorite of kids and adults in all echelons of society. Explore the different options we provide here and create your own muffin melt du jour. Of course, you can replace the muffin with a bagel, pita, or toast.

MAKES 2 MUFFINS, 4 HALVES

Muffin #1—Mediterranean Pesto
2 muffins, halved

½ cup Pesto (page 246)

1 large tomato, sliced thinly

4 artichoke hearts, diced

8 kalamata olives, sliced

½ cup grated vegan mozzarella

Muffin #2—Arugula–Red Onion
2 muffins, halved

2 tablespoons olive oil

Handful of fresh arugula or basil leaves

1 tomato, sliced thinly

4 thin slices red onion

½ cup grated vegan mozzarella

Muffin #3—Kids' Pizza
2 muffins, halved

½ cup pasta sauce

½ cup grated vegan mozzarella

1. Preheat the oven or toaster oven to 350°F. Assemble your muffins in the order that the ingredients are listed.
2. Top with the cheese and bake until the cheese melts, about 10 minutes.

Variations
- For a cheese-less muffin, leave out the mozzarella and sprinkle liberally with nutritional yeast.
- You can also use one of the cheese sauces from the Cheesy Broccoli recipe (page 232) or the Nacho Cheese Sauce (page 242).

If You Have More Time

Use homemade Tomato Sauce (page 101) on Muffin #3.
Replace the mozzarella with cashew cheese (see page 291).

FRUIT AND CREAM CHEESE QUESADILLAS

Most kids will enjoy the sweetness of the fruity filling, and bigger kids enjoy the way the jam melds with the savory cream cheese. Most tortillas are of such a consistency that no oil is needed in the pan to brown them. Still, if you long for that "grilled" flavor, you can coat the outsides or the pan with vegan butter or your favorite oil.

SERVES 2

4 whole-grain flour tortillas
Strawberry or other sugar-free fruit preserves
Vegan cream cheese
1 medium-size banana, sliced very thinly
Vegan butter or oil for cooking (optional)

1. Lay out all four tortillas. Spread the jam over two of them, leaving a 1-inch margin all around the edge (the jam will heat up and start spreading out). Spread the cream cheese over the other two tortillas. Place a layer of banana slices over the cream cheese, pressing them in a little bit, then lay the whole thing on top of the jam tortillas.
2. Heat in a skillet over medium heat (with or without some vegan butter) for about 3 minutes on each side, or until lightly browned. Slice into eight triangles and serve immediately.

Quicker and Easier

Cucumbers are your friend when it comes to a quick and easy snack. You don't need to peel the organic varieties. Slice one up, then top with a splash of freshly squeezed lime juice and a pinch of cayenne and sea salt. You can also top it with a bit of vegan cream cheese and an olive. Another version is to liberally sprinkle with Gomasio (page 278).

Cherry tomatoes are equally versatile. Simply cut off the top portion and follow the above ideas.

MOCHI PIZZETTAS

A popular food in Japan, mochi is a fun and tricky ingredient to work with. It's made from sticky rice and comes in a variety of flavors. It gets puffy when you cook it, and adds a unique, chewy, and crunchy texture to your pizzettas that is sure to stimulate some conversation. They will never come out looking the same way twice. Sometimes they look almost like lava flowing out of a volcano. If you wish for civilized-looking pizzettas, you can shape them using a paring knife or small cookie cutter once they cool a bit. It is possible to make the tomato sauce and still complete the recipe within 30 minutes, although your favorite pasta sauce will do in a pinch.

SERVES 4 TO 6

1 (12.5-ounce) package mochi, thawed
½ cup Homemade Tomato Sauce (page 101) or store-bought pasta sauce
¼ cup grated vegan mozzarella
½ cup diced, seeded bell pepper (go for yellow, red, and orange if available)
Crushed red pepper flakes (optional)

1. Preheat the oven to 450°F and oil a baking sheet well. If you are making the Homemade Tomato Sauce, see page 101 for instructions and prepare it now. Cut the mochi twice crosswise and three times lengthwise to yield twelve pieces. Place on the prepared baking sheet as far apart as possible, bake for 8 minutes, and remove from the oven.
2. Using the back of a spoon, press down the mochi, forming as much of an even surface as possible. It's okay if they are a little Picasso-esque, they will taste just as good. Place a small amount of sauce on each piece of mochi, top with the grated cheese and diced bell pepper. Bake for 5 minutes. Top with crushed red pepper flakes, if desired.

continues

Tips and Tricks

Grainassance makes several mochi flavors, typically in the frozen section of your local health food store. Use the savory varieties for this recipe. If you like the mochi but wish for a thinner crust, you can cut the block in half, reserving half for a later use. Cut the other half once crosswise and twice lengthwise to create six small squares. Take those squares and slice the thickness in half, resulting in twelve pieces that are half as thick.

Variations

- Replace the tomato sauce with Pesto (page 246) and top with a little arugula, diced tomatoes, and diced kalamata olives.
- Instead of creating a pizzetta, you can top the mochi with vegan cream cheese and jam for a sweeter, still hearty, snack.
- For a dessert version, try topping with dark chocolate chips and serving with the Strawberry-Rhubarb Sauce (page 61).

If You Have More Time

Replace the mozzarella with macadamia or cashew cheese (page 291) and add salt to taste. You could also try replacing the tomato sauce with Pesto (page 246).

You can also use one of the cheese sauces from the Cheesy Broccoli recipe (page 232) or the Nacho Cheese Sauce (page 242).

HOMEMADE TOMATO SAUCE

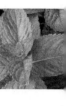

You, too, will be saying, "that's amore" with this quick and easy tomato sauce. It's especially good during the summer, when tomatoes and fresh herbs are abundant. If you have more time, let this simmer over low heat and cook longer, for maximum flavor. We list the tomato paste as optional for those wishing to minimize packaged goods. It definitely enhances the flavor of the dish as well as thickens the sauce.

MAKES APPROXIMATELY 1 QUART

2 tablespoons olive oil

1½ cups chopped yellow onion

4 large garlic cloves, pressed or minced

4 cups chopped tomatoes

1 6-ounce can tomato paste (optional)

3 tablespoons minced fresh basil

1 tablespoon minced fresh Italian parsley

1 teaspoon dried oregano

½ teaspoon dried thyme

1 tablespoon balsamic vinegar

1 teaspoon agave nectar or Sucanat

Sea salt and black pepper

Crushed red pepper (optional)

1. Place the olive oil in a medium-size pot over medium-high heat. Add the onions and garlic, and cook for 2 minutes, stirring frequently.
2. Add the tomatoes and lower the heat to medium. Cook for 5 minutes, stirring occasionally.
3. Lower the heat to low, add the remaining ingredients, and cook for 10 more minutes, stirring occasionally.

Variations
- Additional herbs, such as 1 teaspoon of minced rosemary, 2 teaspoons of marjoram, or 1 teaspoon of fennel seeds, can create a deeper flavor.
- For a heartier sauce, add ½ pound of crumbled extra-firm tofu when adding remaining ingredients.
- For a smoky taste, replace the tomatoes with two 15-ounce cans of fire-roasted tomatoes, or grill your own (see page 28).
- For a **vegan Bolognese** sauce, add 8 ounces of finely chopped tempeh when adding the remaining ingredients. For **Sloppy Joes**, serve the bolognese sauce in a whole-grain bun.

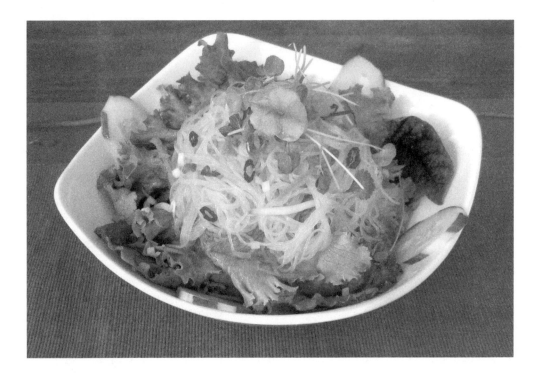

CHAPTER 6

Uplifting Lunches—
Wraps, Rolls, Bowls,
& More

T his chapter highlights some of the all-stars of the quick and easy vegan
lunch: wraps, bowls, and sandwiches. If you prefer to have your largest
meal of the day at lunch, with a lighter meal at dinner, consider this your
dinner chapter.

The beauty of these dishes is that you can quickly combine your favorite ingredients to create a satisfying meal. Since they lend themselves to infinite variations,
rumor has it that you can create a different wrap or bowl every day and never have
the same meal twice.

The wraps and sandwiches are ideal meals on the go. You can create them before leaving your home, or pack up the separate components and assemble them
at your destination. It's also fun to have a wrap night where family and friends can
design their own dish.

Create your own designer bowl by choosing different grains, greens, and protein such as beans, tofu, or tempeh. It's the most frequent meal we enjoy at our
home, especially when combined with a large salad. Give 'em a try and you may
discover that you, too, are drawn to this simple form of dining.

RICE NOODLES WITH MIXED GREENS

When you know you need to eat some leafy greens but you want a little more than that, this is the dish for you. It's a salad with an Asian noodle stir-fry effect. This is low-fat, bursting with flavor, and full of vegetables with the extra fun of rice noodles.

MAKES 2 LARGE BOWLS

4 ounces uncooked rice stick noodles

2 tablespoons brown rice vinegar

2 tablespoons agave nectar

1 tablespoon peeled and minced ginger

2 garlic cloves, pressed or minced

¼ cup soy sauce

1 tablespoon diced red chile, or ½ teaspoon cayenne (optional)

3 cups organic mixed greens or thinly sliced Swiss chard   .

1 medium-size carrot, grated (1 cup)

¼ large cucumber, cut into thin half-moons

Handful of sunflower or mung bean sprouts

2 tablespoons thinly sliced green onion

½ cup minced fresh cilantro

½ cup minced fresh Italian parsley

¼ cup minced fresh mint

Sea salt

1. Cook the rice noodles according to the package instructions.
2. Combine the vinegar, agave, ginger, garlic, soy sauce, and chile, if using. Whisk well.
3. Place the greens, carrots, cucumber, sprouts, green onion, cilantro, parsley, mint, and salt in a bowl and toss with half of the vinegar mixture. Toss the rice noodles in the remaining vinegar mixture.
4. Layer the noodles down on the plate or bowl first and top with the vegetables. If you are storing this dish for later, it would be a good idea to add only enough dressing to the noodles as needed to keep them moist, so they won't get sticky. The rest should be stored separately from the vegetables, or the greens will become soggy and wilted.

Variations

- Experiment with other flavors for this dish by substituting freshly squeezed lime juice for the brown rice vinegar or basil for the parsley.
- Any combination of your favorite vegetables would also be good in this dish. Sautéed mushrooms, eggplant, and zucchini are but a few suggestions.
- Top with toasted sesame seeds for an extra yummy crunch.

Wraps 101

For the uninitiated, there are two or three components to every wrap. The first component is the filling, or that which is wrapped. The second is that which wraps that which is wrapped, or the wrapper. The third and optional component is the sauce in which the wrap may be dipped, or which may be poured or spread in the wrap itself. Make sense? If not, pretend you are at a Chinese restaurant and choose one item from column A and one or more from column B and column C.

These are but a few suggestions. Let your imagination run wild as you design your own innovative and delectable wraps. Of course in many instances, you can use this same method to create a sandwich instead of a wrap, using slices of bread or a bun.

Wraps Demystified		
Wrap	**That Which Is Wrapped**	**Sauce/Spread**
• Flour tortilla* • Nori sheet • Lettuce • Swiss chard • Collard green	• Mixed vegetables (raw, sautéed, roasted, grilled) • Salad Greens • Tofu Scramble (page 62) • Taco Filling (page 228) • Grilled tofu or tempeh • Live Pâté (page 112) • Seed or Nut Cheese (page 291) • Rice and/or beans • Toasted sesame, pumpkin, or sunflower seeds	• Pesto (page 246) • Hummus (page 108) • BBQ Sauce (page 123) • Balsamic Dressing (page 144) • Salad Dressings (Chapter 6) • Garlic-Herb Aioli (page 290) • Salsa (page 82) • Guacamole (page 88) • Tapenade (page 286) • Vegan Sour Cream (page 289) • Vegan Mayonnaise (page 288)
*Many varieties of whole-grain flour tortillas are available, in all shapes and sizes. We like to use the largest ones possible. Try some of the flavored tortillas that are now on the market, such as sun-dried tomato, spinach, and garlic.		

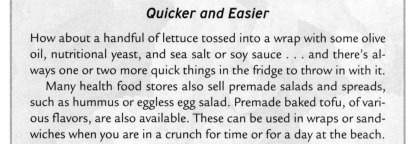

Quicker and Easier

How about a handful of lettuce tossed into a wrap with some olive oil, nutritional yeast, and sea salt or soy sauce . . . and there's always one or two more quick things in the fridge to throw in with it.

Many health food stores also sell premade salads and spreads, such as hummus or eggless egg salad. Premade baked tofu, of various flavors, are also available. These can be used in wraps or sandwiches when you are in a crunch for time or for a day at the beach.

CRUNCHY SALAD WRAP

Wrapping salads in a tortilla is a clever way to eat a good amount of whole foods without feeling as if you are just being too darn healthy. (Yes, it can even get annoying to take care of yourself everyday.) So wrap it up and make it feel like any normal meal. We confess that we like cucumber slices on the side, instead of potato chips.

SERVES 2

---

2 large whole-grain flour tortillas

2 tablespoons sesame seeds

1½ cups sliced green-leaf lettuce

1 medium-size carrot, grated
(about 1 cup)

¼ cup thinly sliced red cabbage

¼ medium-size beet, grated (¼ cup)

1 cup sunflower sprouts
(or sprouts of choice)

¼ cup chopped fresh Italian parsley

¼ cup chopped fresh cilantro

A few thin slices of red onion

1–2 tablespoons olive oil

2 teaspoons nutritional yeast, or to taste

½ lemon

Soy sauce

Sea salt and black pepper

Mustard or prepared salad dressing
(optional)

1. Heat the tortillas in a skillet over medium heat until toasted on each side. Transfer to plates and add the sesame seeds to the hot skillet. Toast for 3 to 5 minutes, or until the seeds are golden brown, shaking the pan occasionally while you begin chopping the vegetables.
2. Prepare all of the vegetables and divide them in half, piling them on top of the tortillas. Add the sesame seeds and your desired quantities of olive oil, nutritional yeast, lemon juice, soy sauce, salt, pepper, and mustard, if using (or any other condiments you prefer). Wrap it up and enjoy. You may wish to use the longer, frilly toothpicks to keep the wraps together for presentation.

If You Have More Time

Although we like to just top our wraps and salads with what is on hand, such as olive oil, lime juice, nutritional yeast, sea salt, black pepper, and Gomasio (page 278), you may want to jazz up your meal a bit more. Try any of the salad dressings from chapter 7 or one of the sauces that are scattered throughout the book.

MEDITERRANEAN HUMMUS WRAP

Hummus wraps are the backbone of quick vegan lunches. Hummus, made from gar-banzo beans (also called chickpeas), is a staple in Middle Eastern cuisine. Here in the West, we tend to fancy up our hummus with everything from sun-dried tomatoes to curry. This bare-bones recipe gives you the foundation you need to make any number of variations. Use it as a filling for wraps or sandwiches or as a dip for crackers or crudités.

MAKES 4 WRAPS

4 whole-grain flour tortillas

1 recipe Traditional Hummus (recipe follows)

8 leaves romaine lettuce, chopped

1 tomato, sliced

½ cucumber, cut into half-moons

½ cup pitted kalamata olives, chopped

½ cup grated carrot (optional)

1. Prepare the hummus according to the directions in the following recipe.
2. Lay out the tortillas, spread with your desired quantity of hummus, and top with lettuce, tomato, cucumber, olives, and carrot, if using. Fold in the sides toward the center, roll it up, and enjoy!

Variations
- If you have more time, you can add Pesto (page 246), cashew cheese (see page 291), or Balsamic Dressing (page 144).

TRADITIONAL HUMMUS

MAKES 1½ CUPS

1 (15-ounce) can garbanzo beans
2 tablespoons tahini
1 tablespoon olive oil
1 tablespoon freshly squeezed lemon juice
1 tablespoon water
2 garlic cloves
¼ teaspoon sea salt
2 teaspoons soy sauce

1. Process all of the ingredients in a food processor until well combined. You may wish to add more water, for a thinner consistency. Start with 2 tablespoons at a time.
2. It is possible to just mash the garbanzos up with a fork if you do not have a food processor, then add all of the other ingredients for a chunkier hummus experience.

Variations

- For a richer version, omit the water and add an extra tablespoon of olive oil.
- For an Italian flair, add four soaked and drained sun-dried tomatoes and ¼ cup of basil leaves, before processing.
- Feeling more Mediterranean? Stir in ¼ to ½ cup of diced kalamata olives and 2 tablespoons of minced fresh Italian parsley after processing.
- Omit the regular garlic and add four cloves of roasted garlic (see page 20), to create a deeper garlic flavor.
- For a garden herb variation, add 1 cup fresh herbs of choice, such as rosemary, cilantro, basil, Italian parsley, sage, marjoram, and thyme, before processing.
- Spice it up by adding a seeded jalapeño pepper and 1 teaspoon of chipotle chile powder, before processing.
- Add a roasted red pepper (see page 21) before processing.

If You Have More Time

Summer Rolls

1. Fill a shallow pan half full with warm water. Place a rice paper sheet in the water and remove within a few seconds. Lay it on a clean surface. We found it's easier to create a summer roll if you use two rice papers per roll. Lay a second soaked paper sheet above the first one with about 2 inches of overlap

2. Place a small amount of chopped lettuce, grated vegetables, and herbs in the center of the bottom rice paper. Fold the sides toward the center and roll up. The rolls should be thin and tightly rolled. Place in a container and cover with a clean, slightly moist towel until ready to serve.

Slice diagonally and serve with Spicy Peanut Sauce (page 193).

Experiment with different veggies (such as carrots, beets, shaved fennel bulb, shiitake mushrooms, or green onion) and herbs (such as parsley, basil, and mint), or grilled tofu or tempeh (page 28), cut into thin strips.

D.L.T.

Dulse is the D. of the D.L.T. A type of seaweed that you can find in most health food stores, it imparts a salty, "taste of the sea" flavor to dishes. Usually dulse is sold as flakes to sprinkle over food, and also as long strips in its original state. You are likely to find it in the Asian foods section. The most common brand is a wild Atlantic variety from the coast of Maine. When toasted, dulse becomes crispy and resembles bacon in appearance—grease-free bacon of course.

SERVES 2

¼ cup lightly packed dulse

4 slices whole-grain bread or
bread of choice

4 leaves romaine or butter-leaf lettuce

4 slices tomato

1–2 tablespoons Vegenaise or
other vegan mayo, or Garlic-Herb Aioli
(page 290), or to taste

1. In a toaster oven, first toast the bread and set it aside. Then, spread the dulse over the toaster oven tray (see Tips and Tricks). You can bake it or just press the toast button, standing by, ready to pull it out when the edges are browning and the strips are getting crisp. It doesn't take long and will probably burn in less than one toast cycle.
2. The rest is standard sandwich etiquette. Dress the toast with Vegenaise; layer with the dulse, lettuce, and tomato; and serve immediately.

Tips and Tricks

You may also heat the dulse on the stove top over medium heat until crispy, being careful not to burn it. Depending on the type of pan you use, you may need to coat it with a little bit of oil.

If You Have More Time

If you happen to crack open a coconut with medium-soft meat, try scooping it out and roasting in a toaster oven at 350°F with a splash of soy sauce, until the edges start to brown, about 10 minutes. You can use this as a substitute for the dulse in this recipe.

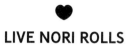

LIVE NORI ROLLS

Nori rolls are convenient for meals on the go or as an elegant appetizer. You can serve them with a simple soy sauce for dipping or with the Spring Roll Dipping Sauce (page 308). Nori sheets come either toasted or sun-dried. Use the sun-dried version for a truly raw roll. The key for a successful raw nori roll is for the pâté not to be too moist or the nori sheet will get soggy and spoil everyone's fun. Here we provide two pâté recipes, each of which lends itself to numerous variations.

SERVES 4

1 recipe pâté (recipes follow)

4 nori sheets

2 cups mixed salad greens

1 avocado, sliced thinly

4 long strips peeled and seeded cucumber (optional)

1 cup grated carrots and/or beets (optional)

1 cup sunflower sprouts (optional)

1. Prepare the pâté according to its recipe.
2. Place a nori sheet, the shiny side down, on a bamboo rolling mat or a clean cutting board. Spread about ¼ to ½ cup pâté on the nori sheet, leaving about 1½ inches at the top of the sheet. Add a small amount of mixed greens, top with a couple of thin slices of avocado, cucumber, grated carrot and beets, and sunflower sprouts, if using. The more fillings you add, the more challenging it will be to roll, so first-timers may want to start with a very small amount and work their way up.
3. Fill a small bowl with water. Begin to roll the nori as tightly as you can, being careful not to tear it. Dip your fingers in the bowl of water and moisten the top 1½ inches of nori. Finish the roll and let it sit, sealed side down, for a few minutes.
4. You can serve the roll in one piece, make a diagonal slice in the center and serve two pieces, or go a step further and cut the halves in half to create four slices per roll. This last way lends itself to creative displays for appetizers or platters.

Note: If the pâté is watery, you can strain out some of the liquid with a cheese-cloth before using in the rolls.

Variations
- Replace the pâté with Macadamia Ricotta (page 219) or another nut cheese (see page 291).
- Adding a layer of Pesto (page 246), or cashew or macadamia cheese (see page 219) on top of the pâté creates an enticing visual, as well as an additional taste sensation!

PEPITA PÂTÉ

Pepita is the Spanish word for pumpkin seed: a dark green seed with a deep, nutty flavor. If you have time to soak them for an hour before using, it improves the flavor. This recipe also works well with sunflower seeds.

MAKES 1½ CUPS

1½ cups pumpkin seeds

1 garlic clove

½ cup water

2 tablespoons freshly squeezed lime juice

2 tablespoons minced fresh cilantro

2 tablespoons nutritional yeast (optional)

2 teaspoons olive oil (optional)

½ teaspoon chile powder

½ teaspoon sea salt, or to taste

⅛ teaspoon black pepper, or to taste

½ teaspoon Nama Shoyu, or to taste (optional)

½ jalapeño pepper, seeded (optional)

1. Soak the pumpkin seeds in 3 cups of water for 5 to 10 minutes. Drain and rinse well.
2. Place in a food processor with the remaining ingredients and process until smooth. You may need to add more water, depending on the strength of your processor. The consistency should be smooth but not watery. Let the mixture sit for 10 minutes or longer before serving, to allow the flavors to marinate.
3. The pâté will last for 3 days when stored in a glass container in the fridge.

Variations

- Replace the pepitas with sunflower seeds or almonds.
- Replace the cilantro with fresh basil, dill, or Italian parsley or a combination of your favorites.
- Add 1 cup of finely chopped vegetables to the pâté after processing.

Superfoods for Health

Pumpkin seeds are a highly nutritious addition to your diet. A good source of protein, fiber, and essential fatty acids, they are also high in magnesium and zinc and are reputed to be beneficial for male prostate health.

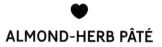

ALMOND-HERB PÂTÉ

Feel free to have fun with different herb combinations and replace the red pepper with a veggie of your choosing, such as celery or red onion. If you want to create an even creamier-textured pâté, and you have more time, you can quickly blanch the almonds according to the method discussed on page 19. Of course you can also use the pâté as a spread on sandwiches or in wraps, or as a dip for crackers.

MAKES 1½ CUPS

1¼ cups almonds

1 tablespoon freshly squeezed lemon juice

1 tablespoon peeled and minced fresh ginger

1 tablespoon olive oil (optional)

½ cup water

¾ teaspoon Nama Shoyu, or to taste (optional)

¼ cup red bell pepper, diced

3 tablespoons minced fresh Italian parsley

1 tablespoon fresh dill

½ teaspoon sea salt, or to taste

⅛ teaspoon black pepper, or to taste

Pinch of cayenne

¼ cup mashed avocado (optional)

1. Soak the almonds in 3 cups of water for 10 minutes, then drain and rinse well.
2. Place them in a food processor with the lemon juice, ginger, water, olive oil, and Shoyu, if using, and process until smooth. The amount of water used will depend on the strength of your processor.
3. Transfer the mixture to a bowl, add the remaining ingredients, and mix well. As with the pepita pâté, this will last for 3 days when stored in a glass container in the fridge.

Variations
- Replace the almonds with walnuts, macadamia nuts, or pecans.
- Replace the parsley and dill with your favorite fresh herbs.
- Replace the lemon juice with lime juice for a subtle change.

Superfoods for Health

Almonds are one of the most healthful nuts around. They are a superior source of plant-based protein, with one ounce of almonds providing close to 6 grams. Almonds are also high in vitamin E and calcium. Enjoy them in almond milk or pâtés, or on their own as a nutritious snack.

MONK BOWL

The Zen simplicity of this dish gives it its name. This is Mark's favorite meal to prepare and a staple at our home. This bowl of enlightenment will hone your multitasking abilities. You can look at this as a three-part symphony consisting of a protein, a grain, and a green. The variations are endless, especially when you begin to add different sauces. Try it with BBQ Sauce (page 123), Spicy Peanut Sauce (page 193), Vegan Sour Cream (page 289), or Enchilada Sauce (page 237).

SERVES 4

1½ cups uncooked quinoa

3 cups water or vegetable stock

1 pound extra-firm tofu

2 tablespoons soy sauce

1 tablespoon coconut oil or other oil

2 tablespoons water

8 cups assorted mixed vegetables—try broccoli, carrots, zucchini, cauliflower, and other favorites

Flax oil or oil of choice

Nutritional yeast

Soy sauce or sea salt

1. Preheat the oven or toaster oven to 350°F. Place the quinoa in a small pot with 3 cups of water over high heat. Bring to a boil. Lower the heat to a simmer, cover, and cook until all of the liquid is absorbed, about 15 minutes.
2. While the quinoa is cooking, cube the tofu according to the instructions on page 27 and place in a small bowl with the soy sauce, oil, and water. Allow to marinate for 5 minutes, stirring frequently. Place the tofu and marinade ingredients on a baking tray and roast for 15 minutes.
3. While the tofu and quinoa are cooking, take a breath and begin the third part of the symphony. Add about 1 inch of water to a medium-size pot with a steamer basket inside. Turn the heat to medium-high. Cut up your vegetables of choice and steam them until tender, about 8 minutes, depending on the vegetables.
4. Place the quinoa in a bowl, top with the steamed vegetables and tofu, and season with flax oil, nutritional yeast, and soy sauce or sea salt to taste.

Variations

- Replace the tofu with tempeh for a hearty, earthy flavor.
- You can also replace the tofu with beans. Simply heat a can of your favorite (pinto, cannellini, and black-eyed peas work especially well), or reheat pre-cooked beans.
- Replace the quinoa with your favorite brown rice pasta or other noodles such as soba or udon.
- Go to town on your vegetable medley with your favorites. Create a rainbow with broccoli, cauliflower, snow peas, zucchini, carrots, purple cabbage, and or bell peppers. Replace the veggies with a mixed green salad and chopped raw veggies.

If You Have More Time

Replace the quinoa with rice (see page 24).
You can also roast the vegetables (see page 20) or stir-fry them (see page 19).

JAPANESE SOBA NOODLE BOWL

Wasabi and pickled ginger are what gives this dish most of its Japanese flavor. However, you may omit them both if you don't have any on hand and still want a warming, satisfying meal. You can add or substitute any vegetables you like, but the mushrooms do add a special flavor to the broth.

SERVES 2 TO 4

1 (8-ounce) package soba noodles

3 cups sliced cremini mushrooms

½ pound extra-firm tofu, cubed

½ medium-size yellow onion, sliced (about 1 cup)

2 + ¼ cups water

¼ cup soy sauce

1½ tablespoons peeled and minced fresh ginger

2 garlic cloves, pressed or minced

1–2 tablespoons wasabi powder

1 tablespoon arrowroot

1 tablespoon pickled ginger, minced

1 tablespoon agave nectar

1 tablespoon sesame seeds (optional)

1 sheet nori (optional)

2 green onions, sliced thinly

1. Boil about 8 cups of water for the soba noodles. Prepare the noodles according to the package directions. Strain and rinse with cold water to stop the cooking process.
2. Meanwhile, place the mushrooms, tofu, onion, 2 cups of the water, and the soy sauce, ginger, garlic, pickled ginger, and agave nectar in another pot over medium heat.
3. In a separate bowl, whisk the wasabi, arrowroot, and remaining ¼ cup of water. Add this mixture to the vegetables, cover, and simmer for 10 minutes.
4. While the veggies are cooking, toast the sesame seeds, if using, in a sauté pan over medium heat for 4 to 5 minutes, or until they are toasty smelling and light brown. Also, use kitchen scissors or a sharp knife to cut the nori sheet, if using, into quarters, then into thin strips.
5. Either add the soba noodles to the vegetables and broth, or keep them separate, ladling the veggies over the noodles. Sprinkle the green onion as well as the nori strips, and sesame seeds, if using, on top. Serve immediately.

Variations

- If you do not favor mushrooms, you can replace them with an equal amount (or combination) of zucchini, carrot, celery, or even sweet potato.
- Replace the tofu with seitan or tempeh.

Tips and Tricks

Before dropping the soba noodles into the boiling water, be sure to remove any wrappers. They are usually wrapped together in three or more little bundles inside the package. If you drop them in without removing the wrapper, they instantly start fusing together. Since soba noodles are so sticky, it is good to stir them up well with a fork when you first put them into the boiling water. Stir them up so well that they are all mixed up and lying in different directions. This will prevent large clumps of noodles.

UDON BOWL

This is a chop-as-you-cook kind of recipe. There are suggested veggies below, but you should feel free to add whatever you like. We like to use celery seeds in our broths, they give a little more of a stock taste. The mushrooms also help to add depth to the flavor of the broth, along with the garlic and ginger, of course. You can serve this dish with as much or as little of the broth as you like.

SERVES 2 TO 4

4 ounces uncooked udon noodles

4 cups water or vegetable stock + water, for boiling udon

1 cup thinly sliced cremini or shiitake mushrooms

1 cup extra-firm tofu, cut into ½-inch cubes

½ cup thinly sliced leek

¼ cup thinly sliced carrots

½ cup snow peas, cut into thirds

1 cup sliced bok choy

¼ cup hijiki or arame

1 teaspoon minced garlic

1 tablespoon peeled and minced fresh ginger

2 tablespoons soy sauce

1 teaspoon miso paste

¼ teaspoon sea salt

⅛ teaspoon celery seeds

¼ cup chopped fresh Italian parsley

2 tablespoons thinly sliced green onion

1. Boil water in a medium-size pot, for the udon. Cook the noodles for 5 to 6 minutes, only until just al dente, as they will continue to cook when you put them in the hot broth later. Strain and set aside.
2. Meanwhile, start heating the water in a medium-size pot over medium-high heat. Chopping as you cook, add the mushrooms, tofu, leek, carrots, snow peas, bok choy, hijiki, garlic, ginger, soy sauce, miso, sea salt, and celery seeds. Bring to a boil, cover, and simmer for 5 minutes.
3. Add the parsley, cooked noodles, and green onion. Serve hot. If you are taking this dish to go, store the noodles separately and reheat them together.

SEITAN CURRY BOWL

Here is another simple variation on the bowl recipes. There are several brands of seitan (a wheat gluten product); you can also look online for instruction on how you can make it yourself. This dish also uses thin rice noodles available in the ethnic food section of most markets. If you don't have any on hand, you can replace them with the pasta of your choosing.

SERVES 4 TO 6

1 tablespoon sesame oil

1 cup yellow onion, chopped small

3 large garlic cloves, pressed or minced

6 shiitake mushrooms, halved

8 ounces seitan, chopped

1 (14-ounce) can coconut milk

1¼ cups water

1½ cups assorted chopped vegetables,
such as broccoli, carrots, and cauliflower

1 small hot pepper, seeded and diced (optional)

1 tablespoon pure maple syrup

2 teaspoons curry powder

1 teaspoon ground cumin

½ teaspoon powdered turmeric

Cayenne

3 tablespoons soy sauce

2 ounces uncooked vermicelli noodles or mung bean threads

2 tablespoons minced fresh cilantro

1. Heat the oil in a medium-size pot over medium-high heat. Add the onion, garlic, and mushrooms, and cook for 2 minutes, stirring frequently. Add the seitan, coconut milk, and water.
2. Add the veggies and cook for 5 minutes, stirring occasionally. Add the remaining ingredients except the noodles and cilantro, and mix well.
3. Add the noodles and cook for 5 minutes, or until all of the vegetables are tender. Add the cilantro and enjoy.

Variation
- Try adding 2 tablespoons of almond or peanut butter along with the coconut
  milk.

QUESADILLA

A staple in households across Mexico, this works best if you have a cast-iron or sauté pan that fits the tortilla, or you may use a griddle. Be sure not to overload the quesadilla with too much cheese or ingredients, to ensure even melting and for keeping the ingredients inside. This is a popular snack for kids, who may just want the cheese and tomato, depending on their finickiness level. You can top with Guacamole (page 88) and/or Salsa (page 82), and Vegan Sour Cream (page 289).

SERVES 4

Vegan butter or oil of choice

4 large whole-grain flour tortillas
(6- to 8-inch)

1 cup grated vegan mozzarella

2 cremini or other mushrooms,
sliced thinly

1 tomato, sliced thinly

2 green onions, sliced thinly

4 olives, diced

2 tablespoons minced fresh cilantro

1. Lightly oil a pan or griddle with the vegan butter. Place a tortilla in the pan. Sprinkle ¼ cup of the cheese in the center of the tortilla, top with one-quarter each of all of the ingredients. Fold the tortilla in half. Heat for a few minutes or until the cheese begins to melt.
2. Gently flip the mixture and continue to cook for a few more minutes. Covering the pan helps the cheese melt faster.

Variations
- Create a spicy version by adding sliced jalapeño or habanero peppers.
- Create an Italian quesadilla (is that an oxymoron?) by using pesto, tomatoes, and vegan cheese.
- You can create a large quesadilla by using two tortillas instead of one folded in half. Simply top the first tortilla with a second tortilla after adding your fillings. Gently flip while heating.
- For a sweet version, see the Fruit and Cream Cheese Quesadilla (page 98).

If You Have More Time

Replace the mozzarella with cashew cheese (see page 291), Nacho Cheese (page 242), or the filling from the Stellar Stuffed Mushrooms (page 188).

GRILLED VEGETABLE SANDWICH

This is another dish that is the height of simplicity. It involves the same process as the Grilled Vegetable Salad (page 303), except here we leave the veggies whole and combine them with all of the fixings to create a sandwich or wrap. The Lemon-Herb Marinade imparts a tangy flavor to the vegetables. Enjoy with condiments of your choosing, or with a spread such as Pesto (page 246) or Garlic-Herb Aioli (page 290). To optimize your time, preheat the grill before you begin gathering the ingredients for the recipe.

SERVES 4

1 recipe Lemon-Herb Marinade
(recipe follows)

1 large zucchini, sliced lengthwise
into ¼-inch strips

1 large red bell pepper, seeded and
quartered

1 small yellow onion, sliced into
¼-inch rounds

4 large shiitake mushrooms

4 slices pineapple, optional

4 whole-grain buns, or 8 slices
bread of choice

8 leaves romaine lettuce

8 slices tomato

Ketchup, mustard, or your
favorite condiment

Lemon-Herb Marinade

¼ to ½ cup freshly squeezed lemon juice

½ cup water

¼ cup minced fresh herbs
(try basil, thyme, oregano, and
Italian parsley)

1½ teaspoons Dijon or
stone-ground mustard

½ teaspoon sea salt

¼ teaspoon black pepper

¼ teaspoon cayenne (optional)

1 tablespoon soy sauce (optional)

1 garlic clove, pressed or minced (optional)

1. Preheat a grill. Combine the marinade ingredients in a large shallow dish and whisk well. Place the sliced veggies in the marinade for 5 minutes. If you have more time, the longer the vegetables remain in the marinade, the more of its flavor they will absorb.
2. Remove the veggies and grill, using tongs to flip occasionally, until char marks appear on both sides. Feel free to baste with olive oil while grilling. You may also wish to grill your bun. Return the veggies to the marinade after grilling.
3. Build your sandwich with the remaining ingredients and condiments of your choosing.

Variations

- Replace the Lemon-Herb Marinade with Balsamic Marinade (page 303).
- Instead of grilling, try roasting the veggies with the marinade at 400° F for 10 to 15 minutes (see page 20). You can also try broiling them on high for 5 to 8 minutes, or until tender and browned.
- Include the meat of a coconut with the veggies.
- For a **grilled Portobello sandwich**, replace all of the veggies except the onion with four Portobello mushrooms. Follow the same instructions as above.
- Try serving on toasted sourdough, rye, or an artisan bread, such as olive-rosemary.
- For a grilled vegetable wrap: Replace the bun with a whole-grain flour tortilla.

Quicker and Easier

You may get cravings for lunch meat or other animal products. The good news is that many vegan products replicate the flavor and texture of animal products. Some of the vegan versions of cold cuts can help with cravings and provide a comfort food effect just when you most need it. We definitely put these in the highly transitional category and don't recommend them as part of a regular balanced diet, but Yves and Lightlife put out some good products. Use a whole-grain bread or bun, spread with vegan mayo or cream cheese, top with all of the fixings, and indulge in a sandwich.

BBQ TEMPEH SANDWICH

This BBQ sauce has been receiving rave reviews from countless satisfied customers over the years. Not only does the tempeh make a rockin' sandwich, you can serve the cutlets over quinoa and top with the BBQ sauce. The sauce is quite versatile as well. It is a favorite for dipping Batter-Baked Tempura (page 184) as well as in Monk Bowls (page 114). If you are using sweetened ketchup, adjust the quantity of sweetener added.

SERVES 4

2 tablespoons soy sauce

1 tablespoon water

1 tablespoon olive or coconut oil

2 (8-ounce) packages tempeh, cut into four cutlets

1 recipe BBQ Sauce (recipe follows)

8 slices whole-grain bread or other bread of choice, toasted (optional)

8 leaves lettuce

1 large tomato, sliced

4 red onion slices

BBQ sauce

MAKES 1½ CUPS

1 cup ketchup

3 tablespoons molasses or barley malt syrup, or 2 tablespoons pure maple syrup

½ teaspoon garlic powder

¼ teaspoon liquid smoke

1 teaspoon chile powder (try chipotle)

1½ teaspoons raw apple cider vinegar

2 tablespoons olive oil

3 tablespoons water

1 teaspoon Dijon or stone-ground mustard

1. Preheat the oven to 350°F. Place the soy sauce, water, and oil in a small dish and add the tempeh cutlets. Allow to marinate for 5 minutes, flipping a few times to evenly coat.
2. Place the tempeh and the marinade ingredients on a baking sheet and cook for 5 minutes. Flip, and cook for an additional 10 minutes.

123

3. While the tempeh is baking, prepare the BBQ sauce by combining all of the in-gredients in a large mixing bowl and whisking well. Pour some sauce over the tempeh while it is baking.

4. When the tempeh is finished cooking, place the cutlet on the bread, toasted if you wish, with the remaining ingredients and as much BBQ sauce as you wish. You can store the extra sauce in a glass container in the refrigerator for up to 5 days

Variations

- Replace the tempeh with an equal amount of tofu.
- Try serving on toasted sourdough, rye bread, or an artisan bread such as olive-rosemary.
- Add 1 tablespoon of minced garlic or peeled and minced ginger to the tem-peh marinade.
- For BBQ sauce: if you don't have ketchup, replace it with one 6-ounce can of tomato paste and ¼ cup of water.
- Another tempeh sandwich idea is our famous **Tempeh Reuben**: Prepare the tempeh as above. Create a Russian dressing by combining 1 cup of Vegan Mayonnaise (page 288) with 1 cup ketchup and mixing in a finely diced large dill pickle. Serve on whole-grain bread with sauerkraut and tomato slices.

If You Have More Time

Create a BBQ Burrito, by chopping up the tempeh and combining it with brown rice, beans, and the BBQ sauce in a wrap.

You can marinate the tempeh longer, or overnight, for a deeper flavor.

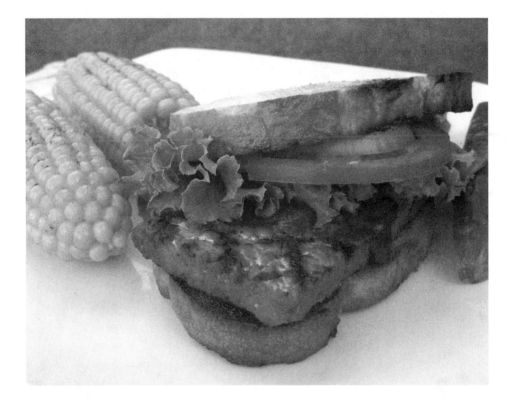

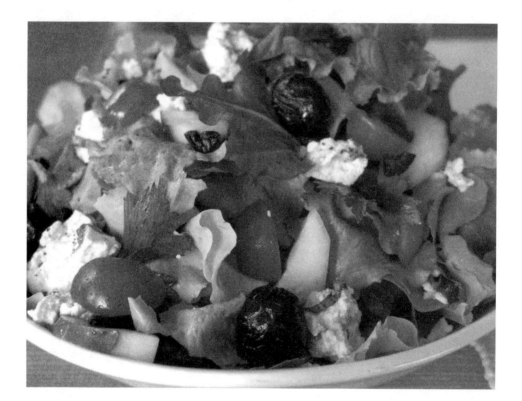

CHAPTER 7

Extraordinary Salads

hile you've heard time and again that eating fresh vegetables and fruits is very good for you, not everyone finds it easy to incorporate them in a yummy way each and every day. We like to think of our food as medicine, and so we create ways to help that medicine go down smoothly, preferably without a spoonful of sugar. The more you grow accustomed to eating a lot of vegetables and fruits, the easier and more satiating they become. Salads are the best way to get a lot of fresh food into your body. Making those salads enticing is what this chapter is all about.

Salads are a cinch to prepare, requiring little technical skill, and yet you can still achieve complex flavors and satisfying meals with them. The Cucumber-Sesame Salad adds a refreshing twist to both Asian and Middle Eastern meals and requires little effort. The Greek Salad with Tofu Feta and the Tuna-Free Tempeh Salad are both perfect examples of salads that do not bore you with simplicity or feel "too healthy." The Vegan Ranch Dressing and Citrus-Curry Dressing can be used to spruce up a simple salad of mixed greens.

This chapter's recipes offer innovative combinations. We're pretty sure nobody will tell you they have already tried a Mexican Salad with Carob Mole Dressing. Most people don't think to make salads out of kale or other greens besides lettuce. How about some fruit in your salad, or nuts, or seeds? Tofu and tempeh, as well as vegetables from the sea, also make for an exotic salad. So live a little as long as you're here and explore the bounty the plant kingdom has to offer.

Salads 101

What can we say? Where would we be without salads? Start with some mixed organic greens and add your favorite veggies. Besides the obvious tomato, cucumber, and red onion, some of our faves include grated beets, carrots, and jicama. Chopped radish or red cabbage adds a pleasant crunch, as do nuts and seeds, either raw or lightly toasted. Avocado is another favorite, as are sprouts of all sorts—try sunflower, buckwheat, clover, and spicy radish.

Turn your salad into a meal by adding beans, cooked grains, roasted or grilled vegetables, or roasted tofu and tempeh cubes (see page 28). The list goes on and on. Create a rainbow of color by adding edible flowers. Some to consider include: onion, chive, basil, dill, chrysanthemum, fuchsias, borage, calendula, chamomile, rose, squash blossom, nasturtium, and more.

Sometimes we make huge salads that are bursting with vegetation, nuts, seeds, and sprouts; so much so that there is hardly any room left for lettuce. Other times it is fun to stick to just a couple of ingredients. Play with your fancy in the moment. Once you have created your masterpiece, here are a few dressings to sample.

VERSATILE VINAIGRETTE

This is a simple recipe from which you can create an infinite array of vinaigrettes depending on what you add to this basic formula. See the variations below for a small sampling.

MAKES 1 CUP

¾ cup safflower oil

¼ cup water

1½ tablespoons raw apple cider vinegar

1 tablespoon freshly squeezed lemon juice

1 tablespoon agave nectar or pure maple syrup

1 garlic clove

2 tablespoons minced fresh cilantro

2 teaspoons soy sauce

Sea salt

Pinch of cayenne (optional)

Place all of the ingredients in a blender and blend until creamy. If whisking by hand, you'll need to press or mince the garlic.

Variations

- For **Italian Dressing**, replace the cilantro with fresh basil and add 1 tablespoon of Italian Spice Blend (page 276).
- Experiment with other oils, such as olive, sunflower, flax, or sesame oil.
- Add 2 teaspoons of Mexican or Indian Spice Blends (page 277).
- Replace the cilantro with other fresh herbs, such as basil, dill, or Italian parsley.
- Try adding 2 tablespoons of pumpkin seeds, sunflower seeds, cashews, macadamia nuts, walnuts, or pecans—raw or lightly toasted (page 26).
- Replace the lemon juice with lime juice or orange juice.

Quicker and Easier

Store-bought dressings are there for you in a pinch. We like the Annie's brand. Feel free to discover your favorites. Keep a bag of prewashed organic mixed greens or organic baby spinach on hand. Toss with some dressing and some beans for a quick and easy salad experience.

CUCUMBER DRESSING

The cucumbers provide abundant liquid and vital nutrients in this low-fat salad dressing. When you desire something light or simply highly nutritious, choose this dressing over the more oil-laden alternatives.

MAKES 1 CUP

1 medium-size cucumber, peeled and seeded (1¼ cups sliced)

⅓ cup soy yogurt

2 teaspoons raw apple cider vinegar or freshly squeezed lime juice

1 teaspoon soy sauce

2 tablespoons chopped fresh mint

¼ cup fresh cilantro

¼ teaspoon sea salt

1 teaspoon nutritional yeast

1 teaspoon balsamic vinegar (optional)

1. Blend all of the ingredients together on high speed for 40 seconds, or until creamy. If you wish to adjust the flavor, allow the dressing to sit for at least 15 minutes first, as the flavor enhances over time.
2. Serve immediately, or store in an airtight container in the refrigerator for 2 to 3 days.

Variation

- ● For a live version, replace the soy yogurt with 2 to 3 tablespoons of chopped macadamia nuts.

CITRUS-CURRY DRESSING

Low-fat, food-based (rather than oil-based) salad dressings are just as satisfying with a fraction of the calories and fat, but high in taste. The ingredients call for foods you might not normally think of as dressing ingredients. Keeping foods like baked squash on hand is a fantastic time-saving habit. This dressing is a superb way to use up that leftover baked squash. This recipe works well with butternut, buttercup, or acorn squash. You can also try it with pumpkin.

MAKES 2 CUPS

1 cup baked squash

2 tablespoons freshly squeezed lemon juice

½ cup freshly squeezed orange juice

1 tablespoon agave nectar

¼ teaspoon sea salt

¾ teaspoon curry powder

½ teaspoon stone-ground mustard

1 teaspoon soy sauce, or to taste

1. If it is necessary to bake the squash, preheat the oven to 450°F, cut the squash in half, discard the seeds, and place cut side down on a baking tray. Add about a ½ inch of water to the pan. Bake it for about 20 to 25 minutes, or until you can easily stick a fork through it. Remove from the oven and allow to cool for a few minutes before scooping some of the flesh out.
2. Blend the squash, along with all of the other ingredients, until totally smooth.

Variation
- Cashews can be substituted for the squash, although they are not low-fat. Start with ½ cup and add more if you desire a thicker consistency.

Quicker and Easier

While we are on the topic of cooked squash, a quick and easy suggestion for serving baked squash is to drizzle it with your favorite oil and top with nutritional yeast and salt. You can mix this in with some cooked quinoa as well, or serve it in a salad. Of course there is the ever-popular drizzling with pure maple syrup and topping with a pinch of cinnamon and nutmeg. A Thai restaurant in our area also serves cooked squash swimming in sweetened coconut milk, as a dessert.

TAHINI-MUSTARD DRESSING

Tahini salad dressings are more of a whole food dressing and are so rich and creamy as well. This is but one flavor variation amongst many. Lemon-Miso Tahini is a big favorite at our home. Like nut butters, the consistency of tahini varies quite a bit from brand to brand, and you'll need to stir the jar well to get a uniform consistency. Otherwise, you'll have oily tahini at the top and rock-hard tahini at the bottom.

MAKES 1 CUP

½ cup tahini

1 tablespoon stone-ground mustard

1 tablespoon raw apple cider vinegar

2 tablespoons soy sauce

½ cup water or more, depending on the consistency of the tahini

Blend or whisk all of the ingredients together.

Variations

- Try replacing the mustard with red curry paste, for a spicy dressing.
- For **Lemon-Miso Tahini** dressing, replace the apple cider vinegar with fresh lemon or lime juice and substitute 1 teaspoon of miso paste for the mustard. For a **Miso-Tahini Spread** for rice cakes, crackers, or sandwiches, leave out the water in the Lemon-Miso Dressing.

VEGAN RANCH DRESSING

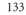

We were surprised to learn that ranch dressing originated from a dude ranch in 1950s California, and that it's actually one of the most popular dressings in the United States. Sometimes you just want to smother your salad in a rich, creamy dressing. This is the one to choose. To turn this into a phenomenal ranch dip or spread, leave out the soy milk.

MAKES 1¼ CUPS

¾ cup Vegenaise, Vegan Mayonnaise (page 288), or other vegan mayo

6 tablespoons soy or rice milk

2 teaspoons freshly squeezed lemon juice

2 teaspoons raw apple cider vinegar

1 garlic clove

2 tablespoons minced green onion, white part only

¼ teaspoon paprika

¼ teaspoon sea salt

¼ teaspoon black pepper

Pinch of cayenne

1 tablespoon minced fresh Italian parsley

1. Blend all of the ingredients except the parsley, until creamy. Pour into a small bowl. Add the parsley, stir well, and enjoy.
2. This dressing will thicken if left in the fridge. Reblend or whisk in some additional soy milk to return it to a pourable consistency.

Variations
- Replace the parsley with an equal amount of fresh dill.
- Add 2 teaspoons of nutritional yeast for a cheeselike flavor.
- For **Green Garden Dressing,** add another tablespoon of minced parsley and include it in the blending step.

ARUGULA, PERSIMMON, AND SNOW PEAS WITH KIWI VINAIGRETTE

The sweetness of the kiwi balances the spiciness of the arugula. Look for the supersweet kiwis to make this dressing a hit. If you're unaccustomed to arugula, feel free to replace some with mixed salad greens. Persimmons are a real treat, when in season. Make sure you use Fuyas, not Hachiyas, which are not ripe until they are too soft to slice. If this delicacy is not available, replace with fresh or dried figs or cherry tomatoes, sliced.

SERVES 4 TO 6

6–8 cups arugula, loosely packed
2 large persimmons, chopped
1 small fennel bulb, sliced thinly and minced
1 large carrot, peeled and grated
2 cups halved snow peas
Sunflower sprouts (optional)

Kiwi Vinaigrette

MAKES APPROXIMATELY 1 CUP

3 kiwis, peeled and chopped (¾ cup)
¼ cup safflower oil
1 tablespoon raw apple cider vinegar
¼ cup water
1 teaspoon agave nectar, or to taste
½ teaspoon Dijon or stone-ground mustard
¼ teaspoon sea salt, or to taste
½ teaspoon soy sauce

1. Combine the salad ingredients in a large bowl. Prepare the kiwi dressing by blending all of the dressing ingredients well. Adjust the amount of agave nectar, depending on the sweetness of the kiwis.
2. Gently toss the dressing with the salad and enjoy.

Variations

- Add 2 tablespoons of toasted macadamia nuts or pine nuts to this salad (see page 26).
- Feel free to add your favorite vegetables, or try adding Pan-Seared Oyster Mushrooms (page 178).
- When persimmons aren't in season, try slicing up a pear, one small mango, or about one-quarter of a pineapple.

Super Foods for Health

Arugula is a somewhat spicy, lemon peppery–flavored dark leafy green. It is a plant-based source of calcium that is loaded with such nutrients as vitamins C, A, and K.

Quicker and Easier

For a quick salad, try 1 cup of halved cherry tomatoes on a small bed of arugula, topped with olive oil, balsamic vinegar, sea salt, and freshly ground black pepper.

WARM SPINACH SALAD

Having organic prewashed spinach on hand makes this dish a whiz to prepare. The unusual delight of a warm salad generates many oohs and aahs from family and friends. We do recommend adding the tempeh bacon to give it an authentic flare.

SERVES 4

4 strips tempeh bacon (optional)
(You can use Fakin' Bacon by Lightlife or
follow recipe on page 57 if you have more time.)
8 cups prewashed spinach, lightly packed
4 cremini mushrooms, sliced thinly
¼ cup thinly sliced red onion
2 Roma tomatoes, thinly sliced into whole circles
1½ tablespoons red wine vinegar
1 teaspoon agave nectar
1½ teaspoons Dijon mustard
2 tablespoons water
½ teaspoon sea salt, or to taste
¼ teaspoon black pepper, or to taste
½ cup chopped walnuts
3 tablespoons olive oil

1. If adding the tempeh bacon or Fakin' Bacon, preheat the oven or toaster oven to 400°F. Place on a baking sheet and bake for 5 minutes. Flip, and bake for another 5 minutes. Remove from the oven and chop into small pieces.
2. Place the spinach in a large mixing bowl with the mushrooms, onion, and tomato.
3. Place the vinegar, agave nectar, mustard, water, salt, and pepper in a small bowl and whisk well.
4. Place the walnuts in a small sauté pan over medium heat and dry-toast for 2 minutes, stirring frequently. Add the olive oil and the tempeh bacon, if using, and cook for 2 minutes, stirring frequently. Add to the bowl with the liquids and mix well. Pour this into the large bowl with the spinach and gently toss well.

Tips and Tricks

Be sure to soak the spinach in water, rinse, and drain well if it's fresh from the market or garden. Dirt has a clever way of attaching itself to spinach and creating a gritty texture that will overshadow the delightful flavors of the dish.

Variations

- Add fresh veggies of your choosing to the salad, such as shaved fennel or diced chile peppers.
- Add green apple slices for a sweet and tart twist.
- Replace the walnuts with pecans or pine nuts.
- You can sauté the mushrooms before adding to the salad. Add them to the pan after adding the olive oil and cook for 3 minutes, stirring frequently.
- Replace the red wine vinegar with balsamic vinegar or your favorite.

If You Have More Time

Add Crunchy Croutons (page 279), Gomasio (page 278), or roasted tofu or tempeh cubes (see page 28) to your salads.

RAINBOW KALE SALAD

Raw kale may seem odd, but once you wrap your mind around the idea, you will be astounded at how delightful it is, especially if you allow time for the dressing to soak in and soften the leaves (see Tips and Tricks). You will soon be out proselytizing its majesty at your next potluck.

SERVES 4

6 cups lightly packed kale, stems removed
¼ cup seeded and diced red bell pepper
¼ cup seeded and diced yellow bell pepper
½ cup grated carrot
½ cup thinly sliced red cabbage

Dressing
2 tablespoons olive oil
1 tablespoon freshly squeezed lemon juice
1 garlic clove, pressed or minced
1 teaspoon pure maple syrup
1 teaspoon soy sauce
¼ teaspoon cayenne

1. Chop the kale and toss in a mixing bowl with the red and yellow bell peppers, carrot, and cabbage.
2. Whisk all of the dressing ingredients together in a small bowl and pour over the salad. Use your hands to massage the dressing into the kale, making sure that it is evenly distributed.
3. Either serve immediately, or chill for 10 minutes or more to allow the kale to soften.

Tips and Tricks

Rubbing oil into the kale and allowing it time to soak in softens the leaves, making them increasingly more palatable with time. Another technique is to quickly toss the kale with a small amount of boiling water, being sure to drain it as soon as the leaves turn bright green (10 to 20 seconds).

Variations

- Although eating a rainbow is recommended for health, don't overconcern yourself with sticking to this precise list of vegetables. Use what you have or what you love.
- Try adding other flavors to the dressing ingredients, such as 2 teaspoons of balsamic vinegar, 1 teaspoon of stone-ground mustard, or ½ teaspoon of red or green curry paste.

Superfoods for Health

Kale is one of our favorite dark leafy greens and is one of the top superfoods in terms of nutrient content and disease-fighting abilities. High in vitamins C, A, and K, it is also loaded with antioxidants, which are known to destroy damaging free radicals.

♥

COLESLAW WITH SHAVED FENNEL

The simplicity of this salad makes it an attractive accompaniment to strong robust entrées frequently found in Indian or even Asian food. When your meal already has enough flavor but needs something fresh and raw, this dish does the trick. The shaved fennel bulb adds a crunchy licorice touch.

MAKES 4 CUPS

1 cup shaved fennel bulb

2 cups shredded green cabbage

1½ cups shredded red cabbage

¾ cup grated carrot

½ cup minced fresh cilantro

¼ cup thinly sliced green onion

2 tablespoons freshly squeezed lemon juice

¼ cup olive oil

1 teaspoon red wine vinegar

2 teaspoons nutritional yeast

½ teaspoon sea salt, or to taste

1. First, cut off any of the stem and herb that may still be attached to the fennel bulb, leaving a flat surface exposing the white concentric layers. You may wish to remove the outside layers if they look dirty. You can use a sharp knife to cut very thin shavings of the fennel bulb, or you can use a vegetable peeler.
2. Mix together the fennel, green cabbage, red cabbage, carrot, cilantro, and green onion in a medium-size mixing bowl. In a measuring cup, whisk together the lemon juice, olive oil, red wine vinegar, nutritional yeast, and salt, and pour it over the vegetables. Mix well and serve, or refrigerate immediately.

Variation
- For a creamier, though not raw, coleslaw, replace the olive oil with Vegenaise, Vegan Mayonnaise (page 288), or other vegan mayo.

CUCUMBER-SESAME SALAD

One of the simplest of salads, this dish is still quite exciting. It's popular with pita bread, on top of salad greens, or alongside Live Hot and Sour Soup (page 155), Batter-Baked Tempura (page 184), or on Sushi Nite (see page 206). If you have a zester, you can use it to grate the nori sheet into ultrafine confetti. Otherwise, the fine side of a cheese grater also works.

SERVES 4 TO 6

¼ cup sesame seeds

4 cups seeded and sliced cucumber, cut ⅛ inch thick
(about 2 large cucumbers)

2 tablespoons thinly sliced green onion

1 tablespoon minced red onion

1 sheet nori, zested or grated finely

½ teaspoon sea salt

2 tablespoons brown rice vinegar

1. Toast the sesame seeds according to the instructions on page 26.
2. Combine with all of the other ingredients in a large bowl, mix well, and serve.

Variation
- For a ♥ live version, do not toast the sesame seeds.

Quicker and Easier

For a simple cucumber salad, try chopped cucumber, sliced tomatoes, and lots of fresh dill. Toss with olive oil and balsamic vinegar or vegan sour cream, and sea salt to taste.

Tips and Tricks

If zesting or grating the nori isn't an option or if it is taking too long, use scissors to cut thin strips. You can cut the nori into 6 long strips, stack 2 or 3 together, and slice again into very thin strips.

SEA VEGETABLE SALAD WITH EDAMAME

Store-bought sea vegetable mixtures usually consist of wakame, akanori, and agar agar. They are similar to the kind of seaweed salads you get at most Japanese restaurants, whereas arame and hijiki are more potent, pungent seaweeds. Serve alongside Live Nori Rolls (page 111), Batter-Baked Tempura (page 184), or on Sushi Nite (see page 206).

MAKES 4 TO 6 SIDE SALADS

2 cups frozen edamame, or 1 (10-ounce) package

Sea salt

½ cup arame or hijiki

1 (½-ounce) package sea vegetable mixture
(we prefer Soken Sea Vegetable Salad)

2 cups shredded green cabbage

½ large cucumber, seeded, cut into half-moons

1 tablespoon brown rice vinegar

3 tablespoons mirin (see Note on page 8 for substitutions)

1 tablespoon toasted sesame oil

2 tablespoons soy sauce

2 tablespoons toasted sesame seeds (see page 26)

1. Bring 4 cups of water to a boil over high heat. Boil the frozen edamame for 5 to 10 minutes, or until they are soft. Strain and sprinkle the hot edamame with sea salt. Set aside to cool. Meanwhile, soak the arame in 1 cup of warm water for 20 minutes, and soak the sea vegetable mixture according to the package instructions.
2. Toss the cabbage, cucumber, brown rice vinegar, mirin, toasted sesame oil, and soy sauce together in a medium-size mixing bowl. Add the edamame and both seaweeds, sprinkle with the toasted sesame seeds, and toss. Serve immediately or store in an airtight container.

Variations

- Try adding 1 teaspoon (or more) of wasabi powder to spice up the mixture. Whisk the wasabi powder together with the mirin and brown rice vinegar so that it blends in well.
- You can also try adding 1 to 2 tablespoons of minced pickled ginger, another Japanese condiment.

If You Have More Time

If you have stores in your area that carry or specialize in Japanese foods, it is fun to design your own seaweed salad blends. Arame, hijiki, and wakame are relatively common forms of seaweed. In most places, akanori and agar agar may be harder to find in their natural form. You may find that seaweed purchased this way is more pungent and needs to be refrigerated if you are not going to use it within three weeks. Have fun discovering the intricacies of the flavors of the sea!

Tips and Tricks

Since many of the nutrients lies just under the skin of a vegetable, we usually do not peel them. For a nice presentation and appealing texture, try using a vegetable peeler to remove stripes of the skin, leaving half of it on. This makes a wonderful compromise.

GREEK SALAD

This salad is truly a meal unto itself. We recommend serving the dressing on the side. The toppings are so pungent that, for some people, very little dressing is desired. If you aren't serving this dish immediately, store the tofu, sun-dried tomatoes, and dressing separately or you are in for one soggy salad.

MAKES 2 LARGE SALADS OR 4 SIDE SALADS

½ pound extra-firm tofu

3 tablespoons freshly squeezed lemon juice (2–3 small lemons)

¾ teaspoon sea salt

6 sun-dried tomatoes, or 1 medium tomato, chopped

6 cups lettuce (green or red leaf, or spring mix), lightly packed

½ cup fresh basil, sliced thinly

½ green bell pepper, julienned

½ medium-size cucumber, halved, seeded, and sliced thinly

¼ cup + 2 tablespoons diced olives (kalamata or green olives)

¼ cup thinly sliced red onion

1 teaspoon capers

Balsamic Dressing
¼ cup balsamic vinegar

¼ cup olive oil

¼ cup water

2 tablespoons pure maple syrup

2 teaspoons soy sauce

½ teaspoon dried thyme

1. In a medium-size bowl, use your hands to crumble the tofu into small chunks that resemble feta cheese. Pour the lemon juice over the tofu and add the salt. Gently stir to coat all of the tofu. Allow to sit either on the counter or in the refrigerator.
2. Soak the sun-dried tomatoes in water to cover and set aside for 20 minutes.
3. Arrange the lettuce on the plates and sprinkle with the basil, bell pepper, cucumbers, olives, onions, and capers.
4. Whisk together all of the dressing ingredients. Transfer to a serving dish or serve right out of the measuring cup.
5. Drain the sun-dried tomatoes and slice into thin strips or dice. Top the salads with the marinated tofu and sun-dried tomatoes, and serve immediately.

Variation

- For a more authentic Greek flair to the dressing, replace the balsamic vinegar with red wine vinegar, replace the maple syrup with freshly squeezed lemon juice, and replace the soy sauce with ½ teaspoon of sea salt, or to taste. You can also add 1 clove of minced garlic, and ¾ teaspoon of dried oregano.

Quicker and Easier

Mark's favorite way to dress a salad is with flax or hemp oil, nutritional yeast, and tamari. Jennifer is content with freshly squeezed lemon or lime juice, nutritional yeast, sea salt, and freshly ground black pepper over hers. You can also go for the well-known basic oil and vinegar dressing—use extra-virgin cold-pressed olive oil and a high-quality balsamic vinegar for a real treat. Quickie salads are another good reason to keep Gomasio (page 278) on hand.

MEXICAN SALAD WITH CAROB MOLE DRESSING

In the United States, mole sauce is usually a savory sauce with a chocolate base. In Mexico, however, the sauce comes in quite a few varieties. Senorita Bombia's Enchilada Casserole, swimming in a divine carob mole sauce, was the most popular dish we served at our restaurant. This salad dressing was inspired out of our love for that far more complicated mole.

MAKES 4 LARGE SALADS OR 6 TO 8 SIDE SALADS

1 (15-ounce) can black beans, or 1½ cups cooked
1 teaspoon soy sauce
2 tomatoes, chopped into medium dice
1 cup corn or thawed frozen corn (optional)
¼ cup minced fresh cilantro
1 cup grated jicama
8 cups salad greens, lightly packed (about ¾ pound)

Carob Mole Dressing
½ cup olive oil
½ cup water
1 tablespoon toasted sesame oil
¼ cup carob powder
1 garlic clove
¼ cup fresh cilantro
1 tablespoon agave nectar
1 tablespoon freshly squeezed lime juice
1 teaspoon soy sauce
1 teaspoon ground cumin
½ teaspoon chipotle chile powder, or
add ½ teaspoon more of regular chile powder
½ teaspoon chile powder
¼ teaspoon ground cinnamon
¼ teaspoon sea salt

1. Drain and rinse the black beans well. Warm them up in a small sauté pan or pot over medium heat with a little bit of water (maybe ¼ cup) and the soy sauce, for about 5 minutes, and strain again. Refrigerate to cool.

2. In a mixing bowl, stir together the tomatoes, corn, and cilantro. Set aside or refrigerate until serving time. Toss the jicama with the salad greens and set aside or refrigerate as well.
3. Blend all of the carob mole dressing ingredients together for 20 to 30 seconds, or until smooth. Transfer to a measuring cup or serving cup, and serve on the side.
4. Add the cooled black beans in with the tomato mixture and stir. Arrange the salad greens on the serving plates. Top with the bean and tomato mixture. Add your desired amount of dressing. Avoid pretossing the salad in the dressing or your precious culinary creation will look brown and unappealing.

Variations
- Replace the black beans with your favorite, such as pinto or kidney beans.
- Use thinly sliced chile peppers to enhance the flavor of the salad. For milder flavor, use poblano, Anaheim, or ancho chile. For some heat, try chipotle, jalapeño, or even habanero (yikes!). Blending one or two into the dressing would also spice things up a bit.

TOFU-GARDEN VEGETABLE SALAD

This colorful variation of our popular "Eggless Egg Salad" lends itself to creative expression as you add your favorite garden veggies and herbs to the tofu base. Enjoy on its own, as a side salad, as a sandwich filling, or as a stuffing in tomatoes or bell peppers.

SERVES 4 TO 6

1 pound extra-firm tofu, crumbled

½ cup diced celery

½ cup diced green onion

½ cup seeded and diced red bell pepper

2 tablespoons diced kalamata olives

½ cup Vegenaise, Vegan Mayonnaise (page 288), or other vegan mayo

1 tablespoon minced fresh dill, or ½ teaspoon dry

2½ teaspoons Dijon or stone-ground mustard

1½ teaspoons raw apple cider vinegar

½ teaspoon minced garlic

1 tablespoon soy sauce

Sea salt and black pepper

1. Combine all of the ingredients in a large mixing bowl and gently mix well.
2. For additional flavor, if you have more time, refrigerate for an hour before serving.

Variations
- Consider adding ½ cup of grated carrots.
- Replace the dill with your favorite fresh herbs.
- For our classic **Eggless Egg Salad**, leave out the bell pepper and olives and add 1 teaspoon of turmeric powder.

TUNA-FREE TEMPEH SALAD

This is a version of Charlie's Relief, one of the most popular dishes from out first cookbook. The name comes from Charlie, the fish mascot of a seafood company. Guess why Charlie is relieved you are enjoying the tempeh version? We had to include it in this book as it has converted so many to believing in tempeh. Serve on its own, with salad, in a wrap or sandwich, or stuffed in tomatoes. Placed on a sandwich with lettuce, tomato, and onion, you will have everyone believing it's the "real deal."

SERVES 4 TO 6

1 pound soy tempeh, quartered

1¼ cups Vegenaise, Vegan Mayonnaise (page 288), or other vegan mayo

⅔ cup diced kosher dill pickles

½ cup diced celery

¼ cup diced red onion

2 tablespoons soy sauce

2 tablespoons minced fresh Italian parsley

1 tablespoon stone-ground mustard

2 teaspoons raw apple cider vinegar

½ teaspoon minced garlic

Black pepper

1. Chop the tempeh into ⅛-inch square pieces. Place in a steamer basket in a medium-size pot and steam for 10 minutes.
2. Remove the tempeh from the steamer basket, combine with the remaining ingredients in a large mixing bowl, and mix well. For additional flavor, if you have more time, refrigerate for an hour before serving.

CHAPTER 8

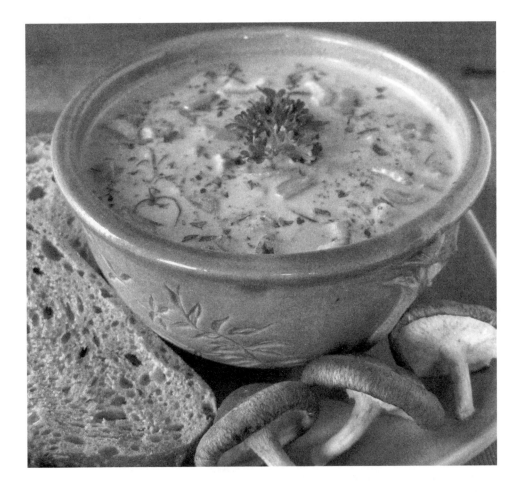

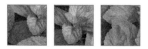

Sumptuous Soups

T his chapter is an example of world cuisine at its finest. Here you will get a chance to travel the globe, visiting Peru, Africa, Mexico, Italy, France, India, and more, through these *30-Minute Vegan* soups. The amount of servings listed in the recipes is based on enjoying these soups as a first course, although many of them can also serve as a hearty meal.

Soup creation is an excellent starting point for introducing folks to quick and easy cooking. The most time-savvy form of soup is a one-pot soup, whereby you simply combine your favorite vegetables in a pot with water or broth, heat until the veggies are cooked, and season to taste. Starting from this humble base, you can experiment with adding different herbs and spices. To this you can add beans, cooked grains, leftover grilled or roasted vegetables, or tofu. Let your imagination be your guide.

Another type of soup is the creamy soup. In vegan food preparation we get the creamy effect by adding nuts, seeds, nondairy milk, or starchy vegetables such as potato or squash to our one-pot soups and blending. You can choose to blend all of the ingredients or blend only some of the ingredients and leave the rest whole to create additional texture.

These recipes call for water or stock as the liquid in the soup. Although we created these recipes with water as a base, you may wish to add some soy sauce or vegetable bouillon to create more depth of flavor. If you have the time, see page 173 to learn how to create your own stock, which will bump up the flavor of all of your soups.

Yes, all of these soups can be prepared within thirty minutes, but if you do have more time, we recommend cooking the soups over a lower temperature for a longer period of time, as this will also enhance the flavor.

Although many people think of warmth when they think of soup, this chapter begins by introducing live soups, those that have not been heated above 116°F. They make use of the flavors present in the raw vegetables and fruits. If you have the time to let these soups marinate for an hour or more, your taste buds will reap the benefits.

♥

LIVE MANGO GAZPACHO

Mangoes make the world go round. That is a scientific fact. Use them to turn your gazpacho up a notch and you will become a chilled soup convert. The flavors will set in more over time so, unless you are serving immediately, don't adjust the seasonings and spices for at least 20 minutes.

SERVES 4

3 cups mango, cut into small cubes (about 3 medium-size mangoes)
(see Tricks and Tips on page 54)

2 cups tomato, chopped small (about 3 medium-size tomatoes)

¼ cup diced red onion

¼ cup minced fresh cilantro

½ red bell pepper, chopped small

1 teaspoon seeded and minced jalapeño (optional)

1 garlic clove, pressed or minced

1 tablespoon freshly squeezed lime juice

1 teaspoon chile powder

¼ teaspoon cayenne

1 teaspoon sea salt, or to taste

1 tablespoon minced fresh Italian parsley

1. Mix all of the ingredients together well in a large bowl.
2. Transfer 2 cups of the mixture to a blender and blend on high speed for 20 seconds and return to the bowl. Mix, and if desired, chill for 30 minutes, otherwise serve immediately.

Variations
- Substitute pineapple, papaya, or additional tomatoes for the mangoes.

♥

LIVE CILANTRO-CUCUMBER SOUP

Ever wonder where the "cool as a cucumber" expression came from? The high water content of cucumbers, and fact that the inside of the cucumber can be a lot cooler than the outside temperature gives this soup a refreshing and cooling effect, a lifesaver on hot summer days.

SERVES 4

4 cups water

1 large cucumber, peeled and chopped (2 cups)

1 cup sliced celery

1 cup chopped avocado

1 garlic clove

2 tablespoons olive oil

2 tablespoons freshly squeezed lime juice

2 tablespoons minced fresh cilantro

¼ cup diced red onion

1½ teaspoons sea salt, or to taste

Pinch of cayenne

1 cup diced jicama (optional)

½ cup diced fennel (optional)

1. Place all of the ingredients except the jicama and fennel, if using, in a blender and blend until smooth.
2. Pour into a bowl and top with jicama and fennel before serving.

Variations
- Replace the cilantro with dill, Italian parsley, or your favorite herb.
- Replace the water with fresh vegetable juice such as Jolly Green Juice (page 37) or Carrot-Vegetable Juice (page 36).

♥

LIVE HOT AND SOUR SOUP

This recipe puts a modern and refreshing twist on the standard Chinese restaurant version of this soup. You may heat it until it is warm to the touch and it will still be considered "live." We prefer using fresh apricots, although dried will do. Figs make a most suitable replacement as well. If you do have more time, the flavor of the soup will improve if you let it marinate for a while, up to a few hours.

SERVES 4 TO 6

2 large shiitake mushrooms

3 tablespoons Nama Shoyu, or to taste

3 cups water

3 fresh apricots, or 5 dried apricots soaked in ½ cup water

1½ cups chopped tomatoes (try Roma)

¼ cup thinly sliced green onion

1 tablespoon peeled and minced fresh ginger

2 tablespoons raw apple cider vinegar

1 jalapeño or other hot pepper, seeded and diced

1 tablespoon agave nectar

2 tablespoons freshly squeezed lime juice

2 tablespoons minced fresh cilantro

½ cup diced cucumber or zucchini

Kernels from 1 ear of corn (optional)

¼ teaspoon cayenne, or to taste

1. Dice the shiitake mushrooms finely and place in a small bowl with the Nama Shoyu to marinate.
2. Place the water, apricots, tomatoes, green onion, ginger, and apple cider vinegar in a blender and blend until creamy. Place in a large bowl with the mushrooms and Nama Shoyu, and the remaining ingredients, and stir well before serving.

Variations
- Replace the water with a vegetable juice of your choosing, such as carrot or carrot, beet, and parsley.
- Replace the cilantro with such fresh herbs as Italian parsley or dill.
- Replace the zucchini with cabbage, bell pepper, carrots, or your favorite raw veggie.

RED ONION SOUP

This uncomplicated soup is quite reminiscent of the more classic French onion soup. If you feel inspired to add a crusty, toasted slice of baguette in there, we're sure you won't regret it. You can also use yellow onions, but the sweetness of the red onions is a special treat. If you don't care for fennel, simply omit it.

SERVES 6

1 tablespoon olive oil

3 medium-size red onions, cut into half-moon slices (6 cups)

4 garlic cloves, pressed or minced

½ teaspoon sea salt

1 cup grated carrot

1 cup thinly sliced celery

2 tablespoons minced fresh tarragon, or 2 teaspoons dried (optional)

½ teaspoon dried thyme

½ teaspoon fennel seed (optional)

½ teaspoon black pepper

¼ teaspoon celery seeds

2 tablespoons soy sauce, or to taste

6 cups water or vegetable stock

2 tablespoons miso paste (preferably dark miso)

6 slices baguette, toasted (optional)

1. Begin to sauté the olive oil, onions, garlic, and salt in a large pot over medium-low heat. Cover while you work on preparing the carrots and celery. Add them to the pot and cover it.
2. Add the remaining ingredients, except the baguette, stirring and re-covering as necessary. Cover and allow the soup to cook over medium heat for 10 minutes, or more if you have time, until the onions are tender.
3. Serve immediately with toasted baguette slices, if desired. Otherwise, allow to cool completely before refrigerating in an airtight container for up to 4 days.

Variations

- Try toasting the baguette covered in a vegan cheese. Then serve with or in the soup.
- Adding 1 cup of thinly sliced fennel bulb would give this soup even more of an enticing flavor.
- Tofu lovers can add up to 1 pound of plain or roasted tofu cubes (see page 28) to the soup along with the vegetables.
- If you cannot get enough greens, add 2 cups of thinly sliced kale or collard greens about 5 minutes before the soup is done cooking.

Quicker and Easier

Miso Soup is the poster child for quick and easy soups. Simply dissolve a tablespoon or two of your favorite miso paste in not quite boiling water. If you wish, you can add diced green onion, minced garlic or ginger, and small cubes of tofu. Top with some shredded nori, season with soy sauce to taste, and you are good to go. Ordinarily you do not boil miso as it destroys some of its valuable nutrients, although it is okay in such recipes as Red Onion Soup because it is being added as a flavor enhancement.

PERUVIAN QUINOA-VEGETABLE SOUP

On our honeymoon in Peru, after politely refusing the house specialty of fried guinea pig, we would typically opt for this yummalicious soup. From the mountains of Cusco to the jungles of the Amazon to the islands of Lake Titicaca, we were happily treated to this national favorite time and time again. Most of these ingredients grow in the Andes Mountains and are popular among the locals. It was amazing to see quinoa growing in its natural environment. If you can't find purple potatoes, any will do.

SERVES 6

7 cups water or vegetable stock

3 tablespoons soy sauce

¾ cup uncooked quinoa

1½ cups chopped purple potatoes, or potatoes of choice

1 large carrot, sliced

¾ cup diced yellow onion

4 large garlic cloves, pressed or minced

1 cup sliced cabbage

1 tablespoon seeded and minced jalapeño or other chile pepper

2 large tomatoes, chopped

¼ cup minced fresh cilantro

¼ cup minced fresh Italian parsley

1 teaspoon sea salt, or to taste

½ teaspoon black pepper, or to taste

1. Place the water and soy sauce in a large pot over medium-high heat. Add the quinoa.
2. Begin prepping the vegetables and place them in the pot as you go. Start with the potatoes, carrot, onion, garlic, cabbage, jalapeño, and tomatoes.
3. Cook until the potatoes are tender and the quinoa is cooked, about 20 minutes from when the quinoa was added. Add the cilantro, parsley, and salt and pepper to taste. Viva Peru!

Variations

- This is an oil-free soup. You may sauté the onions and garlic in 2 table-spoons of olive oil for additional flavor before adding the water, quinoa, and remaining ingredients.
- Add 1 pound of extra-firm tofu, cut into small cubes (see page 27) after adding the vegetables.

Superfoods for Health

Quinoa is perhaps our favorite grain. As one of the easiest and quickest grains to cook, it is definitely the grain of choice for the *30-Minute Vegan*. There are several varieties available including white, red, and even black. High in protein and other nutrients such as lysine, which is good for heart health, it has a delicate nutty flavor. Add cooked quinoa as a side dish to many of the recipes in this book to create a thirty-minute meal. You can start cooking the quinoa before you begin preparation of another dish and within twenty minutes, you will have a nutritious side dish.

ORANGE-BEET SOUP

Served either hot or chilled, this soup is a lighthearted response to its heavier cousin, borscht. Give it a whirl, especially if you are looking for more interesting things to do with beets. If you don't have a zester, you can use the fine side of a cheese grater for the orange zest. Start with ½ teaspoon of zest and increase to 1 teaspoon if desired. Too much zest will make for a bitter soup. A food processor makes quick work of the shredded beets and carrots. Consider serving with a dollop of soy yogurt or Vegan Sour Cream (page 289).

SERVES 6

5 cups water or vegetable stock

4 cups shredded beet (about 3 medium-size beets)

2 cups shredded carrot (about 2 medium-size carrots)

1 cup thinly sliced celery

1 teaspoon sea salt, or to taste

2 teaspoons dried dill, or 2 tablespoons fresh

1 tablespoon miso paste (dark or light)

½–1 teaspoon orange zest (see Tips and Tricks)

1½ cups freshly squeezed orange juice (1–2 oranges)

2 teaspoons pure maple syrup (optional)

1. Start boiling the water and beets over medium heat in a large covered pot while you work on the other vegetables. Add the carrots and celery, covering the pot in between. Add the salt, dill, miso, and orange zest, cover the pot, and simmer for about 5 minutes, or until the vegetables are tender.
2. Remove from the heat, add the orange juice and maple syrup, if using, and carefully blend, in a few batches. The hot liquid will expand in the blender so only fill it a little over halfway, make sure the lid is on tight, and start blending on a low speed if your blender has that option. We like to put a dishcloth over the top for extra protection.
3. Return the blended soup to the pot and reheat if necessary. Serve immediately, or allow it to cool before storing in an airtight container in the refrigerator for up to 3 or 4 days.

Variations

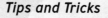

- For a more adventurous flavor, play around with spices. Try adding a pinch of allspice or clove. Or go more savory by adding ½ teaspoon of dried thyme, oregano, or marjoram.
- Adding a few shavings of lime zest also brightens up the brew.
- A sublime topping for this soup is shaved fennel bulb.

Tips and Tricks

You only want to zest the very outside of the orange peel. Don't press down so hard that you get the white pith underneath; this is the very bitter layer. And don't keep zesting away when all of the orange is gone, just to try to get enough zest. This is a common beginner's error, and take it from us, it backfires every time.

Superfoods for Health

A superfood of Russian centarians and reputed to be beneficial for the blood, beets are high in the B-vitamin folate, which is essential for cell maintenance and repair. Look for the firm, unwrinkled ones and wash thoroughly before enjoying. Oftentimes we will leave the skin on organic beets, but always peel the nonorganic. They can be peeled for a brighter color when grating.

PLEASING GREENS SOUP

In San Francisco, where Jennifer lived with her sisters and a couple other wild ladies, this soup was affectionately known as Punishment Soup. Every week before the next delivery of the box of organic food, the ignored and picked-over contents of the box were made into a soup. It became clear that greens were tops on the "I have no idea what to do with this" list. The name soon went to the wayside, however, as a result of everyone's always loving the soup, which led to more and more ideas on how to enjoy all of the greens.

SERVES 4

6 cups water or vegetable stock

4 cups thinly sliced dinosaur kale, lightly packed (also see Variations)

1 yellow onion, chopped

1 cup thinly sliced celery

1 carrot, grated (about 1 cup)

2 garlic cloves, pressed or minced

2 tablespoons peeled and minced fresh ginger

¼ teaspoon celery seeds

½ teaspoon sea salt, or to taste

½ cup minced fresh Italian parsley

¼ cup soy sauce

¾ cup cashews

1. In a medium-size pot over medium heat, combine the water, kale, and onion, and start boiling as you continue to add the remaining ingredients. After everything is in the pot and the mixture comes to a boil, cover, and simmer for 5 to 8 minutes, or until everything is tender.
2. Carefully blend, in a few batches. The hot liquid will expand in the blender so only fill it a little over half way, make sure the lid is on tight, and start blending on a low speed if your blender has that option. We like to put a dishcloth over the top for extra protection. Return the blended soup to the pot and reheat if necessary. Serve immediately, or allow it to cool before storing in an airtight container in the refrigerator for up to 3 to 4 days.

Variations
- Substitute curly kale for the dinosaur kale. Or try a combination of 2 cups of kale, 2 cups of collard greens. Swiss chard also works well but doesn't have as strong a flavor.
- If you have leftover rice on hand, you can substitute it for the cashews.
- You may also substitute a medium-size russet potato for the cashews; simply dice it and add it in the beginning with the kale. Depending on how fast a chopper you are, this may push you over the thirty-minute mark.

MEXICAN TORTILLA SOUP

This Mexican specialty is best enjoyed with a more traditional style of tortilla chip—the kind that are a little thicker than your average chip and supercrunchy. They look more like fried corn tortillas than the more common variety you find in stores, which will get soggy faster in the soup. We offer a recipe to make your own tortilla chips, if you have a little more time and ambition.

SERVES 4 TO 6

1 tablespoon olive oil

1 cup yellow onion, chopped into medium dice

1 Anaheim chile, seeded and sliced thinly

4 garlic cloves, pressed or minced

1 (15-ounce) can diced tomatoes, preferably fire-roasted

1 (15-ounce) can black or pinto beans, drained, or 1½ cups cooked beans

2 teaspoons chile powder

2 teaspoons ground cumin

2 cups water or vegetable stock

2 tablespoons soy sauce

½ medium-size avocado, cubed

¼ cup minced fresh cilantro

2 handfuls of tortilla chips

1. In a medium-size pot, sauté the olive oil, onion, Anaheim pepper, and garlic over medium heat for 3 to 4 minutes, or until the onions are translucent.
2. Add the tomatoes, beans, chile powder, cumin, water, and soy sauce. Cover and allow it to simmer for 10 minutes or so while you prepare the avocado and cilantro.
3. Ladle the soup into bowls and top with a handful of tortillas and a sprinkling of avocado and cilantro.

Variations
- Substitute 1½ cups chopped fresh tomatoes for canned tomatoes.
- Play around with your favorite beans, such as kidney beans, or different varieties of chile peppers such as chipotle, jalapeño, or Serrano.

HOMEMADE TORTILLA STRIPS

Traditionally, the tortillas in this soup are cut in strips rather than triangles. Making the tortillas yourself is worth the effort when you have a little extra time. And you earn some bragging rights. This recipe makes more than you need for the soup because many of them seem to disappear before they hit the table. Although they would traditionally be deep-fried, we prefer the healthier method of simply baking them.

MAKES ENOUGH FOR ONE TORTILLA SOUP RECIPE

2 tablespoons olive oil

6 corn tortillas (usually ½ package)

½ teaspoon sea salt, or to taste

1. Preheat the oven to 400°F. Use a pastry brush to spread a thin coating of the olive oil over both sides of each tortilla. Stack the tortillas and cut them in half, then cut two more parallel lines into each half so that each tortilla is cut into six strips.
2. Oil a baking tray lightly with the olive oil. Lay the tortilla strips on the sheet in a single layer and sprinkle with your desired quantity of salt. Bake for 15 to 25 minutes, or until the tortillas are hard but not browning. They will get crunchier as they cool.

WHITE BEAN–TARRAGON SOUP

White beans and tarragon is a classic food combination—for good reason! Tarragon, an aromatic herb with a licorice-like flavor, is often used in French cuisine. An interesting tarragon tidbit is that the word comes from the French word for "little dragon," due to its root structure. This recipe can serve as a template for many a bean and herb soup. Serve with whole-grain bread.

SERVES 6

5 cups water or vegetables stock

1 small yellow onion, chopped small

1 cup diced celery

4 medium-size garlic cloves, pressed or minced

2 medium-size carrots, thinly sliced

1 tablespoon peeled and minced fresh ginger

¼ cup diced fennel bulb (optional)

2 (15-ounce) cans navy beans, or 3 cups cooked beans

3 tablespoons minced fresh tarragon, or 1 tablespoon dried

2 tablespoons minced fresh chives

2 teaspoons dried thyme

3 tablespoons soy sauce

Sea salt and black pepper

1. Place the water in a large pot over medium-high heat. Add the onions, celery, garlic, carrots, ginger, and fennel, if using, and cook for 10 minutes, stirring occasionally.
2. Add the beans and cook for 10 minutes, stirring occasionally. Remove from heat.
3. Add the tarragon, chives, thyme, soy sauce, and salt and pepper to taste. Stir well and enjoy.

Variations
- Try different bean and herb combinations. Create a Mexican flair with black beans or pinto beans, and fresh cilantro. Go for a Middle Eastern flair with garbanzo beans and Italian parsley. Cannellini beans with basil creates the Italian version.
- Replace the carrots with 2 cups of your favorite garden veggies, chopped small.

continues

- Replace 2 cups of stock or water with vegetable juice of your choosing.
- This is an oil-free soup. If you wish for additional flavor, sauté the onions, celery, and garlic in 2 tablespoons of your favorite oil over medium-high heat for 3 minutes before adding the water.

Quicker and Easier

A wide selection of premade soups is available at your local health food store, which is good when you are absolutely out of time to prepare a meal on your own or for camping trips. Fantastic Foods has several good options. You can liven up these soups by mincing up some fresh garlic or herbs, such as parsley, tarragon, rosemary, or basil. Also, adding fresh vegetables, such as carrots, celery, or kale, will enhance the flavor and nutrition.

INDIAN RED LENTIL DHAL

Dhal is the quintessential dish, served at most Indian meals. Many a yogi are living in the high Himalayas on dhal and rice as their main sustenance. It consists of a legume (typically a lentil or mung bean), Indian spices, and various veggies. Serve this as part of an Indian feast with Coco Rice (page 195), Tofu Saag (page 209), and Chutney (page 287).

SERVES 4

1 tablespoon sesame oil

1 tablespoon cumin seeds

2 teaspoons mustard seeds

1½ tablespoons minced garlic

1½ tablespoons peeled and minced fresh ginger

1½ cups diced yellow onion

1 tablespoon seeded and minced jalapeño or other hot pepper

6 cups water or vegetable stock

1 cup dried red lentils, rinsed well

2 teaspoons curry powder

Pinch of cayenne

3 tablespoons soy sauce, or to taste (optional)

Sea salt and black pepper

3 tablespoons minced fresh cilantro

1. Add the oil to a large pot over medium-high heat. Add the cumin and mustard seeds and cook for 1 minute, stirring constantly. Add the garlic, ginger, onion, and jalapeño, and cook for 3 minutes, stirring frequently.
2. Add the water and lentils, and cook until the lentils are soft, about 20 minutes. Add all the remaining ingredients except the cilantro and cook for 5 minutes. Add the cilantro, remove from the heat, and enjoy.

continues

Variations

- Add 1½ cups of assorted mixed vegetables, such as celery, carrots, zucchini, or your favorite, chopped small, when adding the lentils.
- Try squeezing a lime wedge over your soup and topping with a tad more toasted sesame oil or toasted sesame seeds.
- We like to refer to a bowl of quinoa, covered in dhal and topped with vegan sour cream, as the Mahatma Bowl. If you like an extra kick, hot sauce is another good addition.

If You Have More Time

Become a dhal connoisseur. Replace the lentils with an equal amount of mung beans, or yellow or green lentils. Add more liquid if necessary as the beans cook. To enhance their digestibility, soak the beans overnight. Add salt and/or soy sauce to taste and adjust the other spices, depending on the bean used.

THAI COCONUT SOUP

This soup is most authentic if you can find the kaffir lime leaf, lemongrass, Thai basil, and galangal ginger. Regular ginger and basil will suffice, in a pinch. With the lemongrass, you want to use the softer, bottom white portion of the stalk and be sure to finely mince it. You can also crush the whole stem and place it in the pot at the beginning of the preparation and remove before serving.

SERVES 6

3 cups water or vegetable stock

1 (15-ounce) can coconut milk

3 kaffir lime leaves, or 1 teaspoon lime zest

1¼ cups chopped yellow onion

2 carrots, sliced thinly

3 large garlic cloves, pressed or minced

1 tablespoon peeled and minced fresh galangal ginger

2 cups small broccoli florets

2 cups chopped bok choy

1 tablespoon finely minced fresh lemongrass

1 teaspoon seeded and minced jalapeño or other hot pepper

1 pound extra-firm tofu, small cubes (see page 27)

2 tablespoons freshly squeezed lime juice

1 tablespoon pure maple syrup

1 tablespoon mirin (optional)

2 tablespoons minced fresh Thai basil

3 tablespoons soy sauce, or to taste

1. Place the water, coconut milk, and lime leaves in a large pot over medium heat. Begin prepping the veggies in the order in which they appear above, placing them in the pot as you go.
2. After adding the tofu, allow the soup to cook for 5 additional minutes, or until all of the veggies are just tender.
3. Add the remaining ingredients, remove the lime leaves, and enjoy.

> ### *If You Have More Time*
>
> You can enhance the flavor of the tofu cubes by marinating and roasting them before adding them (see page 28).

SHIITAKE–SEA VEGGIE CHOWDER

Having been raised in New England prohibits us from comparing this dish to that famous chowder. But the similarities as far as warmth, comfort, and satiation are striking. We like to use a large (4½-quart) skillet for making this soup, but any medium-size pot will also do the trick. Cut the veggies small to speed up the cooking process, and keep the flame on low so that you can start the thicker veggies cooking while you're chopping the others, adding them into the skillet as you go.

SERVES 4 TO 6

½ cup arame or hijiki

4 cups water or vegetable stock

1 tablespoon olive oil

2 cups diced russet potatoes, unpeeled

1 teaspoon sea salt

1 teaspoon black pepper

1 cup diced yellow onion (about ½ onion)

1 cup diced carrot (about 1 medium-size carrot)

1 cup diced celery

4 garlic cloves, pressed or minced

4 cups shiitake mushrooms, stems removed, chopped small (about 8 ounces)

½ cup macadamia nuts

2 tablespoons soy sauce

1 tablespoon nutritional yeast

¼ cup minced fresh Italian parsley

1. Soak the arame in 3 cups of water and set aside.
2. Heat the oil, potatoes, salt, and pepper over medium-low heat, stirring occasionally, while chopping the other veggies. Have 1 cup of water on hand and add small amounts to the pan as needed to prevent the potatoes from sticking and burning. Add the onion, carrot, celery, garlic, and shiitakes as you go and keep stirring occasionally until all of the vegetables are soft and tender (3 to 5 minutes after the shiitakes are in). Lower the heat to low.
3. Place the macadamia nuts in a blender and slowly blend while adding 2 cups of the arame soak water (see Tips and Tricks). Blend on high for as long as necessary to grind the macadamias into a milky liquid.
4. Add 1½ cups of the sautéed vegetables to the blender along with the soy sauce and nutritional yeast. Blend for another 20 seconds, or until creamy.

5. Pour the blended mixture back into the sauté pan and add the parsley, arame, and remaining arame soak water, cooking over medium-low heat, stirring, until thoroughly heated. This is a thick soup; heating too long and/or reheating will require you to add a little more water to thin it out.

Tips and Tricks

When making nuts into milks like this one (unstrained), you need to add the water as slowly as possible to make sure that the nuts blend up well. This will be different depending on your type of blender. Too much water will make the nuts (especially macadamia nuts) bounce around in the water and not grind up enough, resulting in chunky milk. Adding the water very slowly in the beginning allows the nuts to form a nut butter consistency, then you can add the remaining water a bit more quickly and you'll have creamy milk.

Variations

- Although the shiitakes lend a very "clamlike" consistency to the soup, you may substitute cremini or other mushrooms when necessary.
- Add a couple strips of diced Fakin' Bacon or Tempeh Bacon (page 57).

Superfoods for Health

Bugs Bunny was on to something. Carrots are a rich source of antioxidants, vitamins, and fiber. Their high level of beta carotene helps improve eyesight. For maximum benefit, enjoy organic carrots regularly in fresh juices. Surprisingly, carrots come in a rainbow of colors in addition to orange. Try yellow, red, purple, black, and white if you can get your hands on them.

AFRICAN SWEET POTATO SOUP

This soup is loaded with flavors that we see a lot in African foods across the land. American's have gleaned many things from African culture, not the least of which is peanut butter. As one of their oldest staple crops, Africans have been making peanuts into butter since ancient times. The peanut was brought to America directly from West Africa. It may be strange to see peanut butter in a soup recipe, but we have made soups for years with this exotic ingredient and pleased many a palate in the process.

SERVES 4 TO 6

6 cups water or vegetable stock

2 medium-size sweet potatoes, cubed (about 5 cups)

1½ cups yellow onion, chopped into medium dice

1 cup thinly sliced carrot

1 cup thinly sliced celery

¼ cup + 2 tablespoons creamy peanut butter

2 garlic cloves

1½ tablespoons peeled and minced fresh ginger

1½ teaspoons ground cinnamon

1 tablespoon ground coriander

¼ teaspoon ground cloves

1 teaspoon curry powder

½ teaspoon crushed red pepper, or to taste

2 tablespoons freshly squeezed lime juice

¼ cup soy sauce

½ teaspoon sea salt, or to taste

¼ cup fresh cilantro, minced

1. In a medium-size pot over medium heat, add 4 cups of the water, and the sweet potatoes, onions, carrots, and celery. Cover, and cook for 5 to 10 minutes, or until the potatoes are tender.
2. Meanwhile, blend the peanut butter, garlic, ginger, cinnamon, coriander, cloves, curry, crushed red pepper, lime juice, soy sauce, and sea salt as much as possible in your blender or food processor. Add 3½ cups of the cooked vegetables and broth, and blend again on high until smooth.
3. Add the remaining 2 cups of water to the pot, and transfer the blender contents to the pot as well. Heat to your desired temperature and allow to simmer for 5 minutes. Add the cilantro when you are ready to serve. If you reheat this soup, you may need to add ½ cup or more of water to get the same consistency.

If You Have More Time

For a simple soup stock, save your vegetable clippings and scraps used in preparing other recipes. Place them in a large, thick-bottomed stockpot over low heat with water to cover and simmer until all of the veggies are completely cooked. Experiment with different vegetables and herbs until you discover your favorite combinations.

Try using onions, potatoes, celery, carrots, parsley, parsnip, zucchini, leeks, and garlic. Many avoid using vegetables that become bitter, such as bell peppers, radishes, turnips, broccoli, cauliflower, greens, and Brussels sprouts. It is not necessary to add dried herbs or spices to a stock. The stock may be frozen and defrosted for future use. You can also pour the broth into ice cube trays, freeze, and use as needed.

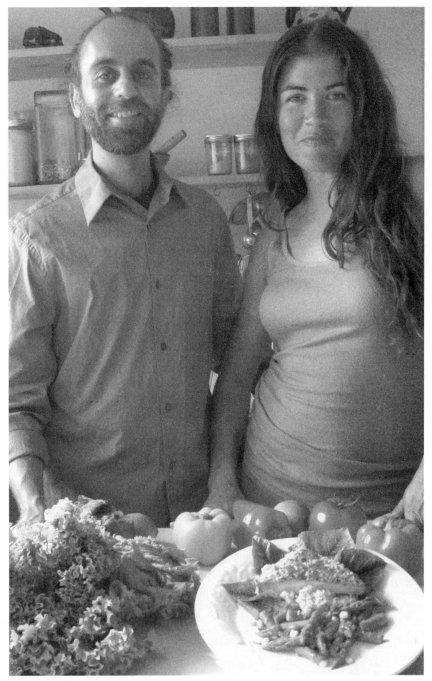

(Photo by Malana Fiore)

CHAPTER 9

Small Plates—
Appetizers, Side Dishes,
& Light Dinners

As serial snackers with a tendency to graze our way through the day, we are big fans of the dishes in this chapter. Therefore we have made it quite simple for you to serve multiple courses without a big time commitment. When you are only cooking for two, it's sometimes hard to tell an appetizer from a main course. Some of these appetizers such as Batter-Baked Tempura, Tofu Satay, or Creamy Asparagus and Toast can be served with a simple salad and called dinner. Most can be served as side dishes with an entrée or soup. All of them make an enchanting first course to one or more of our Wholesome Suppers.

A relatively new style of restaurant for us in the United States is the *tapas* restaurant. Usually of a Spanish influence, these restaurants serve eclectic menus of numerous *small plates,* festive beverages, and spirits like fruit-laden sangria. This style of eating allows you to order a variety of dishes and make a combination that is all your own. Groups can have a lot of fun eating family-style meals with a wide range of options.

As cookbook authors we are rather obligated to provide you with chapters, organization, form, and suggestions. As artists, we are nonconformists at heart and encourage you to be as well. If you want appetizers for dinner, we won't tell anyone. Most of the recipes in this chapter are conducive to a tapas-style meal, so if that's how you want to roll, don't look back.

GINGERED COLLARD GREENS

Asian meets African American! This dish is best when collards are in season in your area. Prepare your ingredients first as you do not want the ginger and garlic to burn, or the collards to overcook. We use tongs to quickly stir the collards while cooking and remove them from the pan while they are still bright green.

SERVES 2 TO 4

1 tablespoon toasted sesame oil

2 tablespoons peeled and minced fresh ginger

2 garlic cloves, pressed or minced

¼ teaspoon sea salt

1½ teaspoons pure maple syrup

6 cups collards, cut into ½-inch strips, loosely packed

1 teaspoon soy sauce

1 teaspoon freshly squeezed lemon juice

1. Place the oil, ginger, garlic, and salt in a medium-size skillet over medium heat. Cook until browning, stirring frequently. Add the maple syrup, and cook for 1 minute more, stirring frequently.
2. Add the collards and soy sauce, and quickly stir (tongs work best for this) for 1 to 2 minutes. Remove from the pan while they are still bright green. Transfer to a bowl and add the lemon juice.

Variations
- Replace collards with other greens, such as Swiss chard or kale.
- Sprinkle with toasted sesame seeds (see page 26).

Superfoods for Health

Collards are one of the most calcium-rich, high-protein greens on the market in a low-calorie package. High in beta-carotene, vitamin C, and soluble fiber, collards are also being studied for their anti-cancer, antiviral, and antibacterial properties.

PAN-SEARED OYSTER MUSHROOMS

This is a simple dish to prepare as a side to many an entrée. Mushrooms are often considered the meat of the plant kingdom (or the fungi kingdom as the case may be). Try this recipe with your favorite mushrooms such as Portobello or shiitake.

MAKES 4 SMALL SIDE DISHES

2 cups oyster mushrooms

2 teaspoons coconut oil or your favorite

1½ teaspoons soy sauce

2 teaspoons mirin (optional)

1½ teaspoons freshly squeezed lemon juice (optional)

Sesame seeds

1. Heat a small sauté pan over medium-high heat. Add the mushrooms and cook until a brown coating is formed, about 4 minutes, stirring frequently. Turn off the heat.
2. Add the oil, soy sauce, mirin, and lemon juice, if using, and stir well for a couple of minutes. Garnish with sesame seeds.

Variation
- For an ultrarich flavor, add a couple of drops of truffle oil with the coconut oil.

Quicker and Easier

Veggie sautés are a quick way to create satisfying side dishes, or tapas. Some of our favorites include asparagus, eggplant, and zucchini. Heat some oil in a sauté pan, add your sliced vegetable, perhaps some minced garlic and a splash of lemon juice. Sauté until just tender, stirring frequently. Add sea salt and freshly ground pepper to taste.

SOUTHWEST ROASTED ASPARAGUS AND CORN

Asparagus is part of the lily family and has been cultivated and revered since ancient Roman times. It comes in three varieties, white, green and purple. This colorful dish works best with thin spears of asparagus. Thicker varieties will require more time. You can also grill the ingredients for an equally delightful experience. Serve as a side dish for any meal, especially Spinach-Herb Stuffed Portobellos (page 204) or Macadamia Nut–Crusted Tofu (page 224). By chance, we discovered this dish makes a superior and unique topping for corn chips.

SERVES 4

1 bunch asparagus, chopped into 1-inch pieces
Kernels from 2 medium-size ears of corn, or 1 (10-ounce) bag frozen
1 large red bell pepper, diced
1 small jalapeño or other hot pepper, seeded and diced
2 tablespoons olive oil
2 tablespoons minced fresh cilantro
1 medium-size lime, juiced
½ teaspoon chile powder
¼ teaspoon ground cumin
Sea salt and black pepper

1. Preheat the oven to 400°F. Place the asparagus, corn, bell pepper, jalapeño, and olive oil in a bowl and mix well. Transfer to a baking sheet and roast until the asparagus is just tender, about 20 minutes, depending on the thickness of the asparagus.
2. Remove from the oven and place in a bowl with the remaining ingredients. Mix well and enjoy.

Variations
- You can create an Italian version by replacing the cilantro and cumin with fresh basil and oregano.
- Try it with specialty chile powders, such as chipotle.
- Try toasting the cumin and chile powder (see page 26).

179

♥

RAWVIOLI PROVENÇALE

Raw Italian food may be a stretch for your imagination, but stretching is a good thing and imagination is the spice of life! So give these little gems an opportunity to impress you with their rich, lovable ways. Serve as an appetizer or side dish along with Raw Pasta Puttanesca (page 202) or as a light dinner along with a drizzle of olive oil, sprinkle of salt, and some minced parsley. For a fancier presentation, serve with Pesto (page 246).

MAKES 16 RAWVIOLIS

½ medium-size zucchini sliced into
thirty-two ⅛-inch-thick round slices

Olive oil

Sea salt

Fresh ground pepper

Minced fresh Italian parsley

Pine Nut–Macadamia Cheese

1½ cups macadamia nuts

½ cup pine nuts

1¼–1½ cups water

1 tablespoon freshly squeezed lemon juice (1 small lemon)

1½ teaspoons raw apple cider vinegar

1 garlic clove

2 tablespoons fresh Italian parsley, packed

1 tablespoon fresh thyme

1 tablespoon fresh rosemary

3 tablespoons nutritional yeast

Sea salt

1. If you do not have a mandoline, use a vegetable peeler to slice thin rounds of the zucchini. It isn't necessary to peel the zucchini. Lay the slices out in a single layer. Lightly brush them with the olive oil, and sprinkle lightly with the salt.
2. Blend all of the cheese ingredients in a food processor for 20 to 30 seconds using only enough water to reach a creamy consistency (too many chunks will rip the delicate noodles). Place 1 heaping tablespoon of cheese onto half of the noodles, place the other halves on top of the cheese and press down a bit.
3. Garnish with a drizzle of olive oil, salt, fresh ground pepper, and some fresh minced parsley.

Variations

- Substitute fresh basil, marjoram, oregano, or other herbs of your choosing for any of the herbs listed here.
- Substitute cashews for the macadamia nuts.
- Substitute cashew cheese for the Pine Nut–Macadamia Nut Cheese (see page 291).
- You can replace the water with rejuvelac if available. This fermented beverage is high in friendly digestive bacteria. It is the strained-off soak water used when sprouting certain grains such as wheat and rye berries. It adds a tangy, cheesy flavor to dishes. (See glossary.)

If You Have More Time

Allow the zucchini noodles, brushed with the olive oil and salt, to sit in the bright sunshine or in a dehydrator set to 145°F for 20 to 30 minutes before assembling them into rawviolis.

Serve with Pesto (page 246) instead of the recommended garnishes.

Serve with Tomato Sauce (page 101).

BRUSCHETTA WITH CROSTINI

Bruschetta has a sort of double-edged sword to it. On the one hand, if you don't make enough of it, it goes so fast and the people want more. On the other hand, you make enough of it, and there is hardly any room for the rest of the meal. Timing is of the essence, try to serve an appetizer like this as close to dinnertime as possible.

SERVES 6 TO 8

3 cups tomatoes, diced (4 to 5 Roma tomatoes)
¼ cup red onion, diced
1–2 garlic cloves, pressed or minced
¼ cup thinly sliced fresh basil
2 tablespoons minced fresh Italian parsley
1 tablespoon balsamic vinegar, or to taste
¾ teaspoon sea salt, or to taste

Crostini
1 baguette, cut into twenty-four ¼-inch slices
1 tablespoon olive oil
1 tablespoon minced fresh parsley, or 1 teaspoon dried
Sprinkle of sea salt

1. Preheat the oven to a high broil. Toss the tomatoes, red onion, garlic, basil, parsley, vinegar, and salt in a mixing bowl and allow it to marinate while you make the crostini.
2. Arrange the slices of baguette on a baking tray or cookie sheet. Use a pastry brush to spread a very light coating of oil onto the bread. Sprinkle the parsley and salt over the bread. Broil for 1 to 2 minutes on each side, until lightly toasted; don't wait for the bread to get brown, or it will dry out as it cools and be too hard to bite through comfortably.
3. Serve immediately or, if necessary, store cooled crostini in a sealable plastic bag at room temperature. They will only last a day or two. Bruschetta will last for 2 to 3 days in an airtight container in the refrigerator.

Variations

- Try using roasted garlic in the bruschetta (see page 20).
- Olive lovers should try adding ¼ cup (or more) of diced olives. The usual brine-cured kalamata and green olives are always good, but lately we prefer the sun-dried oil-cured olives from the Santa Barbara Olive Company for their tart flavor and more interesting texture.
- Mushroom lovers can sauté 2 cups of diced cremini mushrooms in 1 teaspoon of olive oil over medium heat until just soft. Sprinkle with sea salt and add to the bruschetta ingredients.

Quicker and Easier

For a quick **Insalata Caprese Salad**, slice a couple of tomatoes and arrange on a plate with alternating slices of vegan mozzarella. Top with generous amounts of chiffonaded fresh basil, and drizzle with olive oil and balsamic vinegar. Sprinkle with sea salt and freshly ground black pepper to taste. This salad is out of this world when served with garden-fresh tomatoes!

Or go all out and create an **Antipasto Plate** by serving the caprese with mixed olives, artichoke hearts, avocado slices, capers, and sliced pimientos. The truly ambitious could include sliced roasted red pepper (see page 21).

BATTER-BAKED TEMPURA

Here is a far more healthful alternative to the traditional Japanese restaurant tempura, with a light batter that crisps up in the oven. You will want the batter and bread crumbs to be in large bowls with plenty of room for tossing the vegetables around without making a huge mess. You may find this process a bit awkward at first, but with practice, it becomes much easier. We recommend keeping your hands as clean as possible.

SERVES 4 TO 6

2 Portobello mushrooms, cut into ½-inch slices,
or 1 cup cremini mushrooms, halved

2 cups bread crumbs (or pretzel crumbs, see Note)

1 cup broccoli florets

½ yellow onion, cut into ½-inch thick rings

1 cup zucchini, cut into rounds or 4-inch spears

1–2 tablespoons olive oil, for brushing (optional)

Soy sauce for dipping

Batter

3 tablespoons ground flax meal

1 cup water

½ teaspoon baking powder, sifted

1. Preheat the oven to 450°F. Lightly oil a baking tray or cookie sheet. Prepare the vegetables and set aside.
2. Prepare the batter: Blend the flax meal, water, and baking powder for about 10 seconds. Pour the batter into a deep bowl. Place the bread crumbs in a separate deep bowl.
3. Toss the mushrooms around in the batter with a spoon or your hands. Remove them one by one, quickly shaking off the excess batter, and place them in the bread crumbs. When they are all in, swirl the bowl around a bit and use your hands to get them coated in crumbs. Transfer to the prepared baking tray and repeat the process with the broccoli, onion, and zucchini.
4. If you desire crunchier veggies, use a pastry brush to lightly coat oil on the tops of the vegetables. Use a dabbing motion rather than a stroke so as not to brush away the batter (you may even wish to drizzle the oil instead). Bake for 10 to 12 minutes, or until the vegetables are tender.

DIPPING SAUCES

A simple side of soy sauce makes a fine option for your tempura dining pleasure. Still, there are a couple of quick and simple recipes that can enhance your experience. Both make enough for one recipe of Batter-Baked Tempura.

Sweet and Spicy Mustard Sauce
¼ cup stone-ground mustard

½ teaspoon cayenne

1 tablespoon agave nectar or pure maple syrup

Stir together with a spoon.

Classic Tempura Dipping Sauce
¼ cup brown rice vinegar

¼ cup soy sauce

Pour into a bowl and add up to ¼ cup of water, if desired.

Variations
- Substitute any of your favorite vegetables. Carrots, garlic, sweet potatoes, squash, and tofu are all rock-star alternatives.
- For a more exciting dipping sauce add 1 teaspoon of peeled and grated fresh ginger, 2 tablespoons of mirin, and ½ teaspoon of crushed red pepper to the Classic Tempura Dipping Sauce.

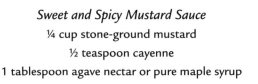

If You Have More Time

Since we could not find any vegan bread crumbs on our little island, we figure some of you may have the same problem. So we whipped up some of our own, using store-bought pretzels—any variety you like will do.

PRETZEL CRUMBS
2 cups pretzels

¼ cup nutritional yeast

2 teaspoons onion powder

1 teaspoon sea salt

2 tablespoons dried parsley

Blend all of the ingredients in a food processor or blender on high speed for 1 to 2 minutes, or until there are very few chunks. Most of it will end up being finer than bread crumbs, which still works quite well.

BAKED PLANTAINS

In Peru, a woman served us bananas, still in their skins, right out of the fire. *¡Que rico!* That simple pleasure was the inspiration behind this dish. Plantains are ripe when they are soft, covered in dark brown spots, and have a slight banana scent to them. The combination of flavors in this dish is surprisingly divine.

SERVES 4

2 large plantains

¼ cup agave nectar

½ teaspoon molasses

½ teaspoon ground cinnamon

1 garlic clove, pressed or minced

1 teaspoon chile pepper, diced, or to taste (optional)

2 tablespoons freshly squeezed lime juice

¼ teaspoon sea salt

½ teaspoon vanilla extract

1. Preheat the oven to 450°F. Bake the plantains, in their skins, on a baking tray or casserole pan, for 20 minutes.
2. Meanwhile, whisk together all of the other ingredients and set aside. Remove the plantains from the oven and set onto a plate to cool for 5 minutes. Remove the peels, cut into ¼-inch slices, pour the dressing over the top, and serve.

Variation
- Substitute bananas when plantains are not available, but don't wait for them to get the brown spots on them, as they may be too ripe for this dish.

CREAMY ASPARAGUS OVER TOAST

In college, Jennifer made a dish much like this one quite frequently, but with far inferior ingredients. The whole-foods approach is much yummier. You can toast any sliced bread for this dish, but if you use an uncut loaf you can have more fun with the shape. Try wedges, tall chunks, stars, or hearts.

SERVES 6

2 tablespoons olive oil

1 cup yellow onion, chopped into medium dice

1 tablespoon minced fresh garlic

2 cups sliced cremini mushrooms (about 8 ounces)

1 teaspoon dried thyme

1 teaspoon black pepper

½ teaspoon sea salt, or to taste

¼ teaspoon celery seeds

1½ pounds asparagus, cut in 2-inch pieces (about 3½ cups)

½–1 cup water

⅓ cup whole spelt flour

2 cups rice milk

6 pieces bread of choice, toasted

Fresh Italian parsley (optional)

1. Sauté the oil, onion, garlic, mushrooms, thyme, black pepper, salt, and celery seeds in a sauté pan over medium heat for 5 minutes, or until the onions are translucent, stirring frequently.
2. Add the asparagus and cover the bottom of the pan with about ¼ inch of water or less. Continue cooking until the asparagus is bright green and just tender. Add water if necessary but the goal is to have the water evaporate.
3. Add the flour and stir for a few more minutes, until the flour starts to brown. Transfer to a blender. You may wish to leave out the tops of the asparagus to add back to the mixture after blending, for texture and appearance.
4. Blend with the rice milk for 30 seconds on high speed until a thick chowder is formed. Return to the pan and heat for 1 to 2 more minutes, while toasting the bread. Serve the chowder over the toast. Garnish with parsley if desired, and the reserved asparagus tops, if using.

Variations
- You can also leave the mixture chunky by using a food processor and pulse-chopping to your desired consistency.

STELLAR STUFFED MUSHROOMS

Always the star of the show, stuffed mushrooms are the quintessential bite-size appetizer. Smaller mushrooms may cook faster, so keep an eye on them. There is more than enough filling here for eighteen large mushrooms. You can be creative with the leftover filling (try using it as a spread over a bagel or baguette). Serve these mushrooms along with Pasta Florentine (page 221), or Macadamia Nut–Crusted Tofu (page 224) and Gingered Collard Greens (page 177).

SERVES 6 TO 8

18 large cremini mushrooms
1 cup spinach, well washed and lightly packed
½ red bell pepper, seeded and roughly chopped
½ green bell pepper, seeded and roughly chopped
2 garlic cloves
½ cup vegan cream cheese
¼ cup nutritional yeast
¾ teaspoon sea salt
¾ cup yellow onion, roughly chopped
1½ tablespoons fresh oregano
1 tablespoon fresh rosemary
½ teaspoon black pepper

1. Preheat the oven to 450°F. Remove the stems from the mushrooms. Place the mushroom caps on a lightly oiled baking tray and place the stems in the food processor along with the remaining ingredients. Blend for 20 seconds, or until a thick, chunky mixture forms.
2. Stuff the mushrooms caps with this mixture and bake them for 15 to 20 minutes, or until the mushrooms are slightly browned. The stuffing will settle as it cools. For maximum flavor and freshness, serve immediately.

Variation
• Replace vegan cream cheese with cashew or macadamia cheese (see page 291).

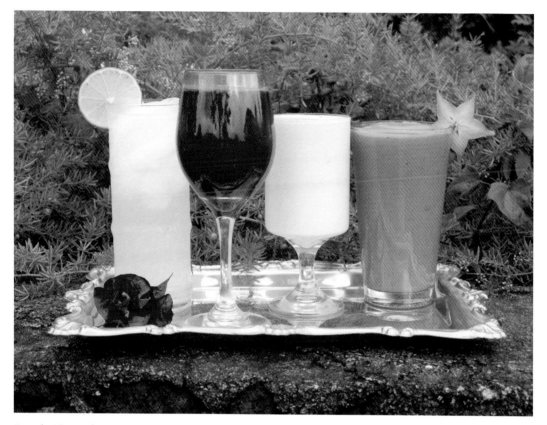

Lovely Limeade • page 38, Watermelon Cooler • page 42,
Basic Nut Milk, Almond • page 42, and Tropical Smoothie • page 47

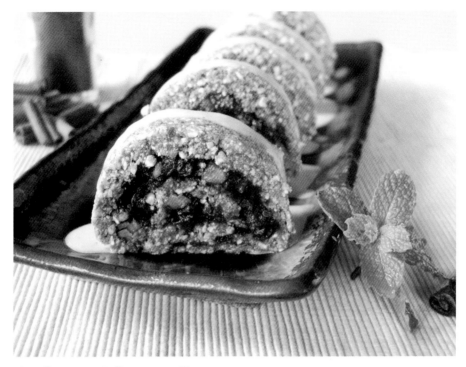

Live Cinnamon Rolls • page 69

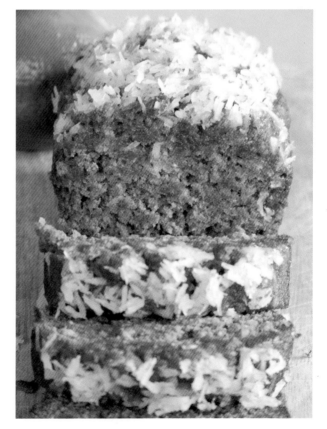

Coconut-Lime
Banana Bread • page 72

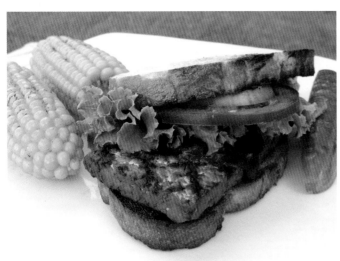

BBQ Tempeh Sandwich • page 123

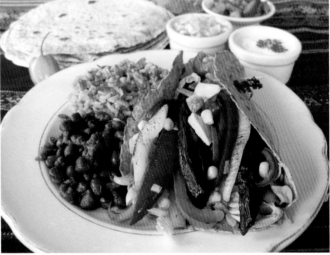

Fajitas Bonitas • page 217

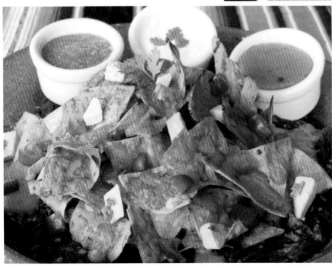

We Will Rock You
Three-Layered Nachos • page 242

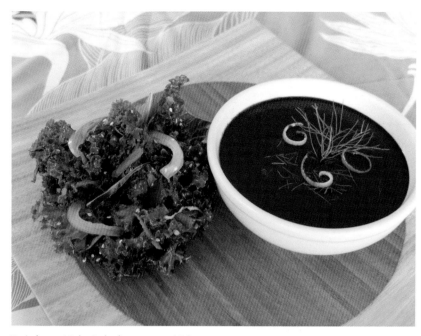

Rainbow Kale Salad • page 138
Orange-Beet Soup • page 160

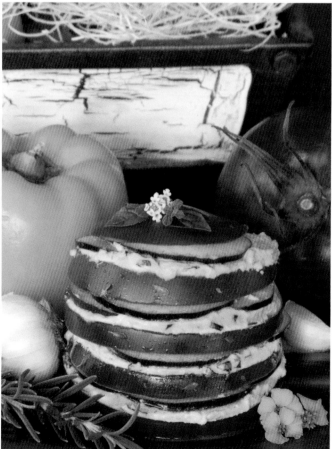

Live Macadamia Nut–Ricotta
Veggie Towers • page 219

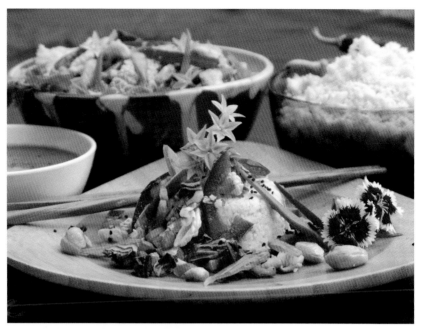

Live Un-Stir-Fry with
Cauliflower Rice • page 198

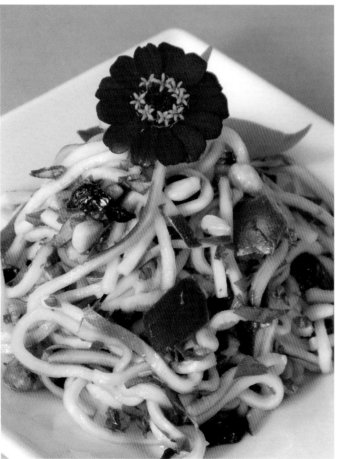

Raw Pasta Puttanesca • page 202

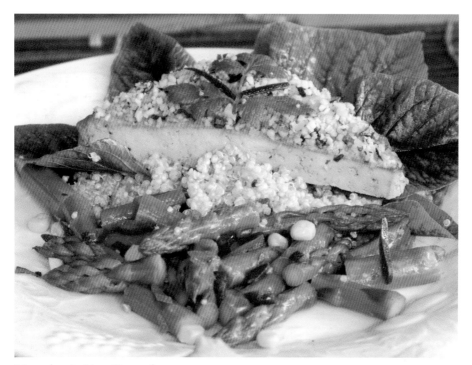

Macadamia Nut–Crusted
 Tofu • page 224
Southwest Roasted Asparagus
and Corn • page 179

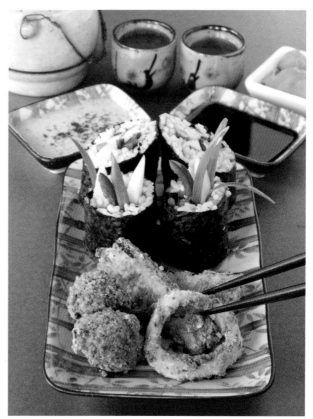

Sushi Nite • page 206
Plain-Jane Roll • page 207
Batter-Baked Tempura • page 184

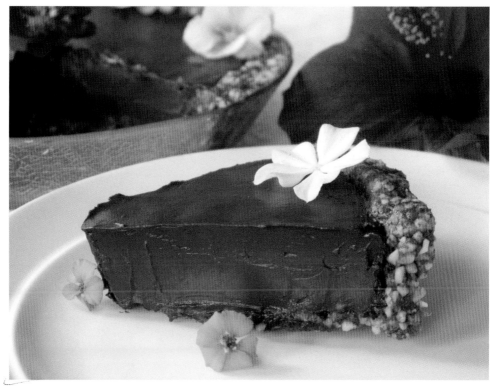
Chocolate Ganache Pie • page 272

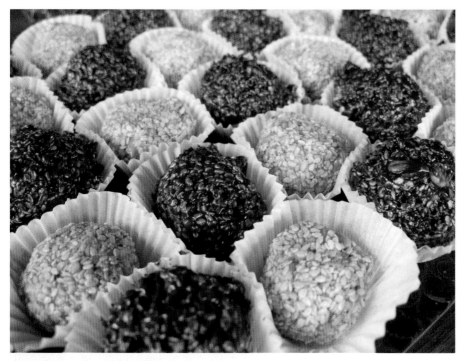
Chocolate-Sesame Bonbons • page 262

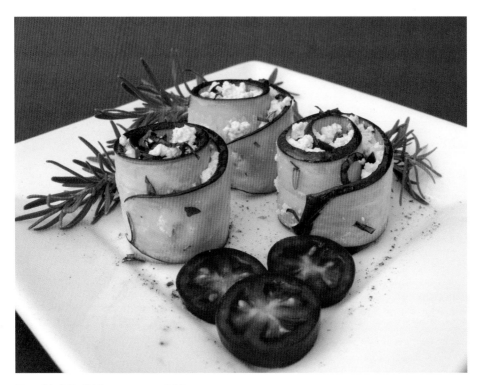

Zucchini Roll-Ups • page 295

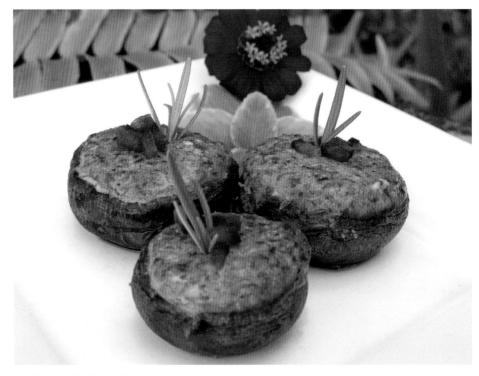

Stellar Stuffed Mushrooms • page 188

JALAPEÑO POPPERS

Out of respect for your arteries, we wanted to create a healthier take on the bacon and saturated fat–filled, deep-fried traditional version. This dish may be a challenge for some to fit into thirty minutes, but it can be done! These are not for the faint of heart; you can adjust the spiciness by how thoroughly you remove the seeds and ribs from the pepper. Be sure to wash your hands thoroughly after handling the jalapeños. Serve on their own or with Salsa (page 82) or Chutney (page 287).

MAKES 10 POPPERS

10 large jalapeño peppers
¼ cup tahini
1 teaspoon soy sauce
3 tablespoons water
¾ cup bread crumbs
(or Pretzel Crumbs, page 185)

Filling
¾ cup grated vegan mozzarella
1 tablespoon vegan cream cheese (optional)
2 tablespoons finely diced red onion
1 teaspoon chile powder
½ teaspoon ground cumin
½ teaspoon sea salt
¼ teaspoon black pepper

1. Preheat the oven or a toaster oven to 425°F. Cut off the tops of the jalapeños. Use a paring knife to remove the seeds and ribs.
2. Place the tahini, soy sauce, and water in a medium-size bowl and mix well. Place the bread crumbs in a separate bowl.
3. Prepare the filling by combining all of the ingredients in a small bowl and mixing well.
4. Lightly oil a baking sheet. Using your hands or a small spoon, scoop the filling into each pepper. Also using a spoon or your hands, spread the tahini mixture onto the peppers and place them on the baking sheet. Liberally pour the bread crumbs over the peppers. Place in the oven and bake for 10 to 12 minutes, or until slightly crispy.

If You Have More Time

If you can't find vegan bread crumbs or want to try another version, try the pretzel crumbs described in the If You Have More Time note for the Batter-Baked Tempura (page 185).

Replace the vegan mozzarella with cashew cheese (see page 291).

Add 1 tablespoon of minced fresh cilantro to the filling.

Add 2 tablespoons of diced Fakin' Bacon or Tempeh Bacon (page 57) to the filling—highly recommended.

POLENTA TRIANGLES

Polenta is a course cornmeal used in Italian cuisine. When cooked, it has a creamy, almost buttery flavor. It's a fun ingredient to work with, especially after it cools, when it can be cut into many creative forms. Admittedly this dish will come very close to the thirty-minute time frame, and will likely go slightly over, unless you are happy to serve the polenta straight out of the oven, without waiting for it to cool. We recommend cooking it in a large pot because it has a tendency to bubble up out of small pots when cooking. You may also wish to wear an oven mitt while stirring, to avoid getting burned. Delish on its own, but if you have more time, top with Pesto (page 246), Tapenade (page 286), cashew cheese (see page 291), or Tomato Sauce (page 101). You can also top the polenta with your favorite grilled or roasted vegetables (see page 20).

SERVES 4

2½ cups water or vegetable stock

1 teaspoon sea salt, or to taste

3 tablespoons thinly sliced leeks or green onion

2 tablespoons minced fresh basil

2 garlic cloves, pressed or minced

¼ cup grated vegan mozzarella (optional)

¾ cup polenta

4 sun-dried tomatoes, soaked in hot or warm water until soft

2 tablespoons soy, rice, or coconut milk (optional)

2 tablespoons nutritional yeast (optional)

¼ teaspoon black pepper

Pinch of crushed red pepper

1. Preheat the oven to 400°F. Place water and salt in a large pot and bring to a boil. While waiting for the water to boil, lightly oil an 8-inch square baking pan or casserole dish. Begin prepping the leeks, basil, garlic, and mozzarella if using. When the water boils, reduce the heat to low and whisk while slowly adding the polenta. Whisk more or less continuously for about 8 minutes. You can take quick breaks to finish up the prepping.
2. Chop the sun-dried tomatoes and add them to the polenta with the remaining ingredients and mix well. Pour into the baking pan or casserole dish and bake for 5 minutes.

3. Remove from the oven. The polenta will begin to solidify as it cools. To fit this recipe into a thirty-minute time frame, place the dish in the freezer for 8 minutes, or until it is firm enough to cut but still warm enough to serve. Cut into four squares and slice each square diagonally, to form eight triangles.

Variations

- Try adding 2 tablespoons of minced kalamata olives and/or chopped artichoke hearts.
- Replace the basil with your favorite minced fresh herbs, such as Italian parsley, rosemary, and oregano.

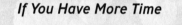

If You Have More Time

Once the polenta is done cooking, you can place it in the refrigerator for 30 minutes or longer until completely firm. Now is the time to break out all of the unused cookie cutters for a creative display. Cut into triangles or desired shapes and grill or sauté before serving. You can also place it on a baking tray and reheat in a 350°F oven for 10 minutes.

Quicker and Easier

There is a fabulous precooked organic polenta available from the Quinoa Corporation that comes in a few different flavors. It's available in most health food stores and is sold in a cylindrical tube. Simply slice into ½-inch rounds and bake, grill, or sauté according to the instructions on the package. Top with pesto, cashew cheese, tomato sauce, herbs, or nutritional yeast, or serve with a salad.

HERBED FLATBREAD

We wanted to create a simple yeast-free bread that would fit into our thirty-minute time frame. The baking time may push this over the thirty minutes, depending upon your chopping speed. Experiment with different herbs, ideally fresh from the garden or market. For the dough, we used whole wheat pastry flour. It will also work with white spelt flour, which will require less water. Start with 1½ cups. The dough consistency should be somewhat moist and elastic. This bread rocks when used for sandwiches, for toast, and as a pizza crust for our Pesto Pizza (page 245).

MAKES ONE 10 X 16-INCH FLATBREAD

5 cups whole wheat pastry flour	1 teaspoon minced fresh rosemary
2 tablespoons baking powder	1 teaspoon minced fresh oregano
1 teaspoon sea salt	1 teaspoon fresh thyme
3 tablespoons minced fresh basil	¼ cup olive oil
2 tablespoons minced fresh Italian parsley	1¾–2 cups water

1. Preheat the oven to 425°F. Well oil an 10 x 16-inch or similar size baking dish. Sift the flour and baking powder into a large mixing bowl. Add the herbs and salt, and mix well. Add the oil and slowly add the water, mixing with a spatula.
2. When all of the liquid is absorbed, begin mixing with your hands, and gently knead the dough for 2 minutes. The consistency should be somewhat moist and elastic. Add more water if necessary.
3. Place on the baking pan and spread an even layer using a spatula, rolling pin, or your hands. Place in the oven and bake until golden brown on top, about 18 minutes.

Variations

- Try adding 1 tablespoon of minced garlic, 3 tablespoons of minced sun-dried tomato and/or 3 tablespoons of minced kalamata olives.
- Replace the herbs with your favorite herbs and spices.
- Try making bread sticks by sculpting the dough on the oiled pan. You may need two pans for this and the baking time will be less—between 12 and 15 minutes, or until lightly browned.

Quicker and Easier

For a quick garlic bread, drizzle or brush olive oil on whole-grain bread or baguette slices, top with minced garlic or garlic powder, and sprinkle with sea salt. You can also use vegan butter for a more buttery effect. Toast as desired.

TOFU SATAY

Traditionally, tofu satay is a popular Indonesian and Thai kebab with a spicy peanut sauce. To fit the recipe into a thirty-minute time frame, serve fondue style, with some fancy toothpicks. You can also serve this as an entrée with Coco Rice (page 195) or quinoa. Use any leftover peanut sauce for a Monk Bowl (page 114) or as a dipping sauce for Summer Rolls (page 109).

SERVES 4

1 pound extra-firm tofu, sliced into 8 cubes (see page 27)

1 tablespoon soy sauce

1 tablespoon toasted sesame oil

1 tablespoon water

1 large red bell pepper, seeded and chopped into 1-inch chunks

2 green onions, sliced thinly

Spicy Peanut Sauce

MAKES 2 ½ CUPS SAUCE

1 (14-ounce) can coconut milk

¼ cup + 2 tablespoons peanut butter

1 garlic clove

1 tablespoon freshly squeezed lime juice

4 teaspoons soy sauce

1 tablespoon toasted sesame oil

1 tablespoon minced fresh cilantro

2 teaspoons pure maple syrup

1 hot pepper or jalapeño, seeded and minced, or crushed red pepper flakes

1½ teaspoons curry powder (optional)

1. Preheat the oven or toaster oven to 350°F. Place the tofu cubes, soy sauce, oil, and water in a small bowl and gently mix well. Allow to marinate for 5 minutes, stirring frequently. Transfer to a well-oiled baking sheet and roast for 20 minutes.
2. While the tofu is marinating and cooking, prepare the peanut sauce by placing all of the ingredients in a blender and blending until smooth. Pour a small amount of the sauce onto the baking tofu as soon as you finish blending it. Pour the remaining sauce into a bowl for dipping.

3. To serve fondue style, place the tofu in a bowl when done cooking and top with the green onion. Place the bell pepper in another bowl. Serve with toothpicks for dipping.

Variations
- Replace the peanut butter with almond butter.
- Replace the tofu with tempeh.
- You can also replace the tofu with seitan. Instead of marinating and roasting, simply sauté one 8-ounce package of seitan in 2 tablespoons of oil and 1 tablespoon of soy sauce over medium-high heat until golden brown, about 5 minutes, stirring frequently.
- For an even more authentic Thai flavor, add to the peanut sauce 1 kaffir lime leaf, and 1 tablespoon of peeled and minced fresh galangal ginger.

If You Have More Time

Create the kebab of your dreams by using your favorite veggies. Try with mushrooms; onions; red, yellow, and orange bell peppers; and cherry tomatoes. Place on skewers with the tofu and place on a baking sheet. Broil on high for 10 minutes. Serve with the peanut dipping sauce.

COCO RICE AND BEANS

Yah, mon, this is a classic Jamaican combination. The key to creating the ideal consistency is to make sure to use the correct quantity of water and coconut milk. Serve with Jamaican Vegetable Medley (page 213), Baked Plantains (page 186), and Gingered Collard Greens (page 177) for a Caribbean feast.

SERVES 8 TO 10

2 cups white basmati rice	1 (14-ounce) can coconut milk
1¾ cups water or vegetable stock	1 (15-ounce) can black-eyed peas, drained and rinsed (1½ cups cooked beans)
1 teaspoon fresh thyme	
½ teaspoon sea salt, or to taste	

1. Place the rice, water, thyme, salt, and coconut milk in a medium-size saucepan over medium-high heat. Bring to a boil. Lower the heat to a simmer, cover, and cook until the liquid is absorbed, 15 to 20 minutes.
2. Remove from heat and transfer to a large mixing bowl with the beans. Gently mix well and enjoy.

Variations

- Leave out the beans and thyme for simple **Coconut Rice.**
- Experiment with different bean and herb combos, such as black beans and cilantro, red beans and Italian parsley, or white beans and basil. Use 2 table-spoons of minced fresh herbs for these variations.
- Add 1 tablespoon of peeled and minced fresh ginger or garlic to the rice while cooking.
- For **Coco Spinach Rice**, replace red beans with garbanzos and stir in one 10-ounce package of frozen spinach or 2 cups of tightly packed fresh spinach, ½ cup of chopped roasted cashews, and 1 tablespoon of curry powder. Add more salt or soy sauce to your liking.
- For a **Sweet Coco Rice**, omit the thyme and black-eyed peas and add 1 medium-size mango, cubed when the rice is done cooking. Serve warm with some coconut milk sweetened with agave nectar.

If You Have More Time

This recipe works well with other grains, such as brown basmati, short or long grain brown rice, and millet. Follow the grain cooking chart on page 24 for quantity of liquid and cooking time. Make sure the coconut milk is counted as part of the liquid.

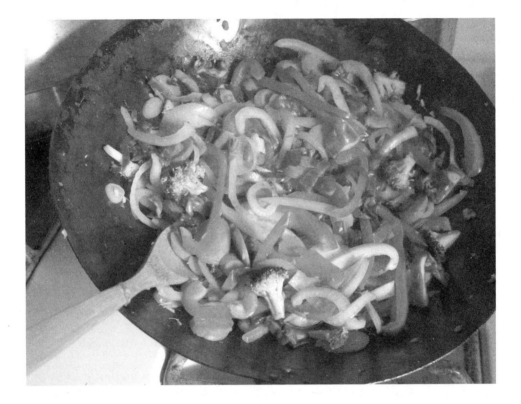

CHAPTER 10

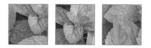

Wholesome Suppers

Enjoying vegan cuisine as the main course often requires a gentle shift in perspective from the typical approach that utilizes plant-based food solely as a side dish. If you've been doing this for some time, you know the benefits. If you're new to vegan foods, it's a shift you will find to be quite rewarding. An immense variety and depth of flavors await you in the form of a vegan centerpiece. This chapter also highlights the world's cuisines, so get ready to experience a bounty of culinary delights from all around the globe.

We selected dishes that range from the super simple, to the more complex. The Tofu Saag and Seasoned Steamed Veggies can easily be completed in less than thirty minutes. Others such as Live Un-Stir-Fry and Macadamia Nut–Crusted Tofu will encourage you to multitask and will reward you with depth of flavor. Please remember that with practice, you will get faster and more creative with your dishes.

Some of the recipes are meals unto themselves, others are for the entrée alone. You will likely wish to prepare one of the many side dishes or appetizers to enhance your meal. You can also create a thirty-minute meal by serving the entrée with a large salad or along with quinoa or pasta, both of which can be prepared while you work on the recipe.

Although frequently a protein such as tempeh or tofu takes center stage, sometimes a hearty pasta or vegetable medley easily fills that role. Our cutting-edge live food entrees feature "pasta" and "rice" that are made from vegetables, and the Veggie Towers are filled with macadamia nut ricotta that rivals the real deal. Have a hungry family or friends to feed? You'll also find recipes for two of our favorite family meals: sushi night and taco night—perhaps they will be a hit in your home as well!

197

♥

LIVE UN-STIR-FRY WITH CAULIFLOWER RICE

Last year, we sponsored the Most Remarkable Vegan Recipe Contest in History. The winner received an all-expense paid trip for two to Kaua'i. We received innovative recipes from all over the country and the world. This is a simplified variation of the winning recipe created by Felix Schoener of Martfield, Germany. One taste and we think you will know why this one's the winner!

SERVES 4 TO 6

Vegetable Medley
2 cups chopped napa cabbage
½ cup chopped red cabbage
½ cup thinly sliced carrots
1 red bell pepper, seeded and julienned
½ cup julienned snow peas (optional)
1 cup thinly sliced shiitake mushrooms
2 tablespoons chopped fresh cilantro
¼ cup thinly sliced green onion
¾ cup cashews

Spicy Vegetable Dressing

MAKES 1¼ CUPS

½ cup sesame oil
3 tablespoons agave nectar or pure maple syrup
2 tablespoons umeboshi plum vinegar or raw apple cider vinegar
3 tablespoons Nama Shoyu
1 small kaffir lime leaf, or zest of 1 lime
1 (½-inch piece) peeled fresh ginger
1 garlic clove
1 tablespoon dehydrated onion flakes
1 teaspoon seeded and diced Thai chile or jalapeño
1 stalk lemongrass, finely chopped (only the bottom part) (optional)
1 tablespoon tamarind paste (optional)
1 teaspoon toasted sesame oil
(optional—leave out for the completely raw version)

Cauliflower "Rice"

4 cups cauliflower florets

½ cup macadamia or pine nuts

½ teaspoon sea salt

1 tablespoon dehydrated onion flakes

½ teaspoon garlic powder

1. Combine all of the vegetable medley ingredients in a large bowl and mix well. Place all of the dressing ingredients in a blender and blend until creamy. Add to the vegetable medley and toss well.
2. Prepare the cauliflower rice by placing all of the ingredients in a food processor and pulse-chopping until a smooth but textured consistency is reached. Do not overprocess or it will get too mushy.
3. Serve the vegetable medley on a bed of cauliflower rice. If you have more time and want to get fancy, you can press the cauliflower into a ring mold for an elegant style of presentation.

Variations

- Add 1½ cups of sliced young coconut or your favorite veggies such as zucchini, cucumbers, bean sprouts, or lightly steamed broccoli to the vegetable medley.
- Add 1½ cups of raw or lightly steamed broccoli to the vegetable medley.
- You can serve the vegetable medley over quinoa or rice.

If You Have More Time

If you have a dehydrator, you can create more of a sautéed vegetable effect by dehydrating the vegetables in the dressing for 30 minutes at 130°F or until warm to the touch. On a bright, sunny day you can also try to place the bowl of veggies in the sunshine, stirring occasionally for 30 to 45 minutes to soften them up quite a bit.

You can also replace the cashews in the vegetable medley with **Spicy Cashews:** Simply combine ¾ cup of chopped cashews (or macadamia nuts or almonds), ½ teaspoon of sesame oil, ½ teaspoon of chile powder (chipotle, if you can find it), ½ teaspoon of onion powder, ½ teaspoon of sea salt, and a pinch of cayenne in a small bowl and mix well.

SEASONED STEAMED VEGGIES WITH QUINOA

Steaming is a quicker, healthier alternative to sautéing your food. And with this mixture of spices and seasonings, you won't feel deprived. If you don't care for fennel seeds, try substituting mustard seeds, or one of your favorite spices.

SERVES 4

1½ cups uncooked quinoa

3 cups water or vegetable stock

2 cups broccoli florets

2 medium-size carrots, cut into thin 4-inch spears

1 large zucchini, halved and sliced ¼ inch thick

½ large yellow onion, chopped

2 teaspoons cumin seeds

2 teaspoons fennel seeds

2 teaspoons dried thyme

1 teaspoon sea salt

2 tablespoons olive oil

2 tablespoons nutritional yeast

2 tablespoons mirin (optional)

1. Bring the quinoa and water to a boil in a medium-size pot, cover, and lower the heat to low. Simmer for 15 to 20 minutes, or until all of the water is absorbed.
2. In another pot over medium heat, place a steamer basket over 1 to 2 inches of water. Start prepping the veggies in the order they are listed: broccoli, carrots, zucchini, and onion. Cover and simmer. You shouldn't have to stir them, when the onions are translucent and you can stick a fork easily into the zucchini, about 5 minutes, remove the pot from the heat.
3. Meanwhile, toast the cumin and fennel seeds in a skillet over medium heat until an aromatic toasty fragrance is emitted. Add to a blender with the thyme, salt, olive oil, nutritional yeast, and mirin, if using. Blend, going from low to high speed, for 15 to 20 seconds, or until the seeds are chopped up well.
4. Toss the vegetables in the seasonings and serve on top of the quinoa.

Variations

- As usual, your favorite vegetables will work just as well here. Potatoes, sweet potatoes, and squash will take 5 to 10 minutes longer to steam. Tofu is another good option to accompany your veggies.
- Trade out the spices or add your preferred flavors. Mustard seeds, caraway, curry powder, and oregano come to mind.
- Substitute your favorite pasta or grain for the quinoa.

Quicker and Easier

Steam up your favorite veggies and season with flax oil, nutritional yeast, and soy sauce to taste. For a simple meal, add tofu cubes to the vegetables while steaming and serve with quinoa.

RAW PASTA PUTTANESCA

Although some people might be skeptical of the concept of raw pasta, this is the sort of living foods entrée that appeals to almost everyone. The abundance of flavor and the heartiness of the dish will distract even the most critical and apprehensive diner. The zucchini noodles will astound you. They are a fantastic gluten-free substitute in any pasta dish. The olives add immense character to this dish, so be sure to purchase a good quality brand. We recommend Santa Barbara Olive Company's sun-dried olives!

SERVES 4

4 medium-size zucchini (8 cups "noodles")
(see Tips and Tricks)
1 tablespoon olive oil
⅔ cup pitted olives, diced
2 large tomatoes, chopped (2 cups)
½ cup minced fresh Italian parsley
½ cup chiffonaded fresh basil
2 teaspoons fresh thyme
4 garlic cloves, pressed or minced
2 teaspoons capers (optional)
½ teaspoon sea salt, or to taste
Black pepper
2 tablespoons pine nuts

1. Prepare the zucchini noodles with a mandoline set to the ⅛-inch julienne setting. Set aside or place in the refrigerator.
2. Add all of the remaining ingredients to a mixing bowl, stir well, and allow to sit for 3 to 5 minutes.
3. To serve, divide the noodles among four plates and top with your desired amount of vegetables, making sure to distribute all of the juices, too. Alternatively, toss the noodles and vegetables together and allow people to serve themselves.

Variations

- For a more transitional dish, prepare the vegetables as instructed but replace the zucchini noodles with spaghetti noodles or pasta of your choice.
- Add some heat to this dish with ½ teaspoon crushed red peppers or 1 teaspoon diced chile pepper of choice.
- Toasting the pine nuts will add a more complex flavor. (see page 26)
- If you have more time, try tossing the zucchini noodles in Pesto sauce (page 246) before topping with the vegetables.
- Olive lovers can feel free to double 'em up.

Tips and Tricks

You do not need to peel the zucchini before noodling them, but choose the flattest side to start on. If you do not have access to a mandoline (see Glossary), you can try using a vegetable peeler. If the zucchini is thick, you may need to slice it in half before it will fit through your vegetable peeler. Peel off as many layers as possible, then slice those layers into ⅛-inch noodles, using a knife. The pile of noodles won't look quite as large if you use the peeler method, so you may wish to account for that with more zucchini or smaller (looking) servings.

We recommend not combining the noodles with the vegetables until you are ready to serve them, as the oil and liquid will start to break down the noodles and reduce them in size.

SPINACH–HERB STUFFED PORTOBELLOS

This dish utilizes fresh bread rather than the more traditional bread crumbs. The bread soaks up the extra liquid from the sautéed vegetables and creates a stuffing-esque topping. Try to get portobellos that have a bit of a bowl shape to them. This way the filling stays in better when you are moving them around. Don't fret if you can only find flat or inverted ones, though, they still taste equally satisfying. Serve on a bed of quinoa or Coco Rice (page 195) if you have more time. You can also serve with Roasted Garlic Mashed Potatoes (page 235) and Mushroom-Onion Gravy (page 236).

SERVES 4

4 large Portobello mushroom caps

3 tablespoons olive oil

1 + 2 teaspoons soy sauce

Four ½-inch slices baguette

6 cups thinly sliced spinach, lightly packed
(about 6 ounces)

½ red bell pepper, seeded and diced

½ yellow bell pepper, seeded and diced

¼ cup fresh basil, minced

¼ cup fresh Italian parsley, minced

1 teaspoon dried thyme

2 garlic cloves, pressed or minced

Sea salt

1. Preheat the oven to a high broil. Remove and discard the stems of the Portobellos and set the caps on a baking tray. Combine 1 tablespoon of the olive oil with 1 teaspoon of soy sauce in a small bowl, and rub or brush the mixture onto the mushrooms. Place them, scales down, on the baking tray and broil for 3 minutes, or until the bottoms are lightly browned. Flip them over and broil again for 2 to 3 minutes, or until the tops are lightly browned. Remove from the oven and set aside.
2. Meanwhile, using 1 tablespoon of olive oil, lightly brush the baguette slices and sprinkle with salt. Place them on their own tray or pan under the broiler for 1 to 2 minutes on each side to brown them lightly. Remove and chop into ½-inch cubes.
3. In a sauté pan, combine the remaining 1 tablespoon of olive oil and 2 teaspoons of soy sauce with the remaining ingredients. Sauté for about 5 minutes, or until the veggies are bright and tender. Turn off the heat, add the

bread, and stir. Top the Portobellos with equal amounts of the filling. Broil for another 3 to 4 minutes, or until everything looks toasty, but be careful not to scorch the bread.

Variations
- Try substituting diced summer squash or zucchini for the bell peppers.
- Substitute Swiss chard, collard greens, or kale for the spinach.
- Add or substitute fresh rosemary, oregano, or tarragon for any of the herbs listed here.
- Replace the bread with small roasted tofu or tempeh cubes (see page 28).

Quicker and Easier

Set the oven to a high broil and oil a baking tray. Slice a medium-size eggplant into ½-inch rounds, and place on the baking tray. Broil for 15 minutes, or until a knife can pass through the center of the eggplant easily. Top with tomato sauce and grated vegan mozzarella.

SUSHI NITE

Admittedly, mastering the art of rolling sushi takes most people a fair amount of practice. If you count the time it takes to prepare the rice, this recipe will go over the thirty minutes. We include these because not only are maki rolls guaranteed to impress your guests but with practice, they get easier and easier to make. You don't even need a bamboo mat, although some people swear by them, to get the roll as tight as can be. We use a little extra water to cook the rice to get that desired sticky consistency. Our other secret to good rice is preparing it early in the morning (perhaps as you get ready for work). Then just leave it sitting on the stove or countertop, covered, until ready to roll. This way the rice will be thoroughly cooled but not hard from being refrigerated.

We offer three varieties of nori roll fillings. In your beginner stage, start with just one filling at a time. It's just as satisfying with less work. The Plain-Jane Roll works for kids (you may want to omit the green onion). These go great served with the Batter-Baked Tempura (page 184), and Miso Soup (see page 157).

MAKES 4 NORI ROLLS

Rice

2 cups brown or sushi rice

4¼ cups water or vegetable stock

1 tablespoons brown rice vinegar (optional)

2 tablespoons mirin (optional)

¼ cup toasted sesame seeds (optional)

1. Bring the rice and water to a boil, cover, and simmer for 30 to 40 minutes, or until the rice is soft and most of the water is absorbed. A little excess water is okay and will make the rice stickier as it cools.
2. If using, add the brown rice vinegar, mirin, and sesame seeds, and stir together.
3. Allow to cool either on the countertop, or, if pressed for time, in the refrigerator. You can still roll with warm rice but you will have to work faster as the heat softens the nori, which will tear while rolling if you wait too long.

Tips and Tricks

If the nori does tear, keep rolling, and then wrap it in another nori sheet. You may want to dab a little water across the second sheet to get it to stick to the first one.

Plain-Jane Roll

½ large avocado

½ cucumber, peeled, seeded

4 stalks green onion, green part only

1 medium-size carrot

Cut all of the veggies in long strips. For the carrots, you can use the vegetable peeler to make thin, easy-to-bite-through strips.

Asian Dream Roll

¼ cup sea veggie salad, soaked for 10 minutes
(we use Soken; to create your own, see page 6)

3 cups shiitake mushrooms, sliced thinly

1 teaspoon toasted sesame oil

1 teaspoon soy sauce

1 tablespoon water

4 stalks green onion, green part only

1 tablespoon pickled ginger

1. Be sure to soak the sea veggie salad first so it is ready to go when you are done with the mushrooms.
2. Sauté the mushrooms, sesame oil, soy sauce, and water over medium-low heat in a small sauté pan for 5 to 6 minutes, or until the mushrooms start to brown, stirring frequently.
3. Meanwhile prepare the green onion and pickled ginger.

Asparagus Roll

8–12 asparagus spears, bottoms snapped off
(see Tips and Tricks)

1 teaspoon olive oil

¼ teaspoon sea salt

¼ teaspoon garlic powder

½ red bell pepper, sliced into long thin strips

½ large avocado, sliced into long thin strips

4 stalks green onion, green part only

1. Boil the asparagus in a sauté pan with ⅓ cup water for 3 minutes to soften. Add the olive oil, salt, and garlic powder, sauté for 3 to 4 more minutes, and remove from the heat.
2. Meanwhile, prepare the red bell pepper, avocado, and green onion.

continues

To roll your sushi

4 nori sheets

¼ cup pickled ginger, or to taste

Wasabi

Soy sauce

1. Fill a small bowl with water. Lay out all four nori sheets on a clean countertop with the long side running parallel to the counter's edge (this gives you longer rolls).
2. Scoop ¾ to 1 cup of the rice mixture onto each sheet. Use your hands, a spoon, or a rice paddle, to spread the rice over each sheet, leaving only a 1-inch strip along the top edge. Dipping your hands in the water will prevent the rice from sticking to you.
3. Clean your hands off and add your preferred filling, lining everything up about 1½ inches from the near edge of the sheet. You can let some of the veggies stick out the ends for an artistic presentation.
4. Grab the near edge and roll it up, using a good amount of pressure to keep the roll as tight as possible. Work quickly so that it doesn't have time to wobble around. Dip your fingers in the water, wet the exposed 1-inch strip of nori, and keep rolling until that edge is on the bottom. Press firmly, and leave it with the seam side down while you move on to the other rolls.
5. When all four are rolled, start with the first roll and transfer to a cutting board. Cut a diagonal line through the middle with a serrated knife, then cut straight lines halfway through each half. Set on plates and garnish with pickled ginger, wasabi, and soy sauce.

Superfoods for Health

Sea vegetables such as the ones found in this recipe have been consumed in Japan and around the world since ancient times. They have the most minerals of any food and are rich in iodine, essential for proper thyroid function. Look for the organic varieties, without added coloring, at your local health food store.

TOFU SAAG

This is a vegan take on a traditional Indian Dish that uses paneer, a type of cheese abundant in Indian cuisine. To prepare a meal in the thirty-minute time frame, use frozen organic spinach and serve with quinoa. For the Taj Mahal of Indian meals, serve with Coco Rice (see page 195), Chutney (page 287), and Red Lentil Dahl (page 167).

SERVES 4

1 pound extra-firm tofu	1 tablespoon curry powder
2½ tablespoons soy sauce	1 teaspoon ground cumin
¼ cup water	½ cup soy, rice, or coconut milk
1 small yellow onion, chopped small	2 teaspoons ground coriander
4 large garlic cloves, pressed or minced	1 teaspoon sea salt, or to taste
1 tablespoon peeled and minced fresh ginger	Pinch of crushed red pepper
1 pound frozen spinach, thawed (2 cups, pressed firmly)	Diced red bell pepper and minced fresh cilantro

1. Preheat the oven or a toaster oven to 350°F and oil a baking sheet well. Cube the tofu (see page 27), and place on the baking sheet with the soy sauce. Allow it to sit for 5 minutes before placing it in the oven. Roast for 15 minutes, and remove from the heat.
2. While the tofu is roasting, place the water in a large sauté pan over medium-high heat. Add the onion, garlic, and ginger, and cook for 5 minutes, stirring frequently. Lower the heat to low, add the spinach, and cook for 5 minutes, stirring occasionally. Add the tofu and the liquid from the baking sheet, and the remaining ingredients, and cook for 5 minutes.
3. Garnish with the diced red pepper and cilantro leaves if desired.

Variations
- Add 1 cup of chopped tomato and/or 1 cup of fresh or frozen peas when adding the tofu.
- Try toasting the cumin (see page 26).
- This is an oil-free dish. If you wish, you may replace the water with 1½ tablespoons of sesame oil for added flavor.

If You Have More Time
Add a medium-size potato, cooked and chopped into ½-inch cubes, and/or 1½ cups of lightly steamed cauliflower when adding the tofu.

THAI GREEN CURRY

Obviously the easiest way to make this curry would be to buy curry paste at the store, in which case we recommend the Thai Kitchen brand. Although it is not organic, the flavor is far better, and stronger, than most. However, if you take a few extra minutes to make your own Thai Curry Paste (page 280), you will be far more pleased and you'll probably impress yourself! You can just as easily make this a recipe for red curry by substituting red chiles for the green.

SERVES 4 TO 6

1 recipe Thai Curry Paste, green option (page 280),
or 2–3 tablespoons green curry paste (see Tricks and Tips)

1 pound extra-firm tofu, cubed
(see page 27)

1 cup thinly sliced carrot

1 red bell pepper, seeded and chopped

2 cups shredded bok choy or green cabbage

1 cup whole fresh basil leaves

1 (15-ounce) can coconut milk

½ cup water

1–2 tablespoons agave nectar (optional)

1 cup mung spouts

1 cup minced fresh cilantro

1. Prepare the Thai Curry Paste according to the instructions on page 280 and place in a large sauté pan or pot over medium heat (see Tricks and Tips if using store-bought curry paste). Add the tofu, carrot, red bell pepper, bok choy, and basil leaves as they are ready, stirring and turning the heat down to low once the mixture is bubbling.
2. Add the coconut milk, water, and agave. Cover and simmer for about 5 minutes, or until the carrots are tender. Add the sprouts and cilantro. Stir and serve.

Tips and Tricks

If you are using store-bought curry paste: Heat 1 tablespoon coconut, sesame, or olive oil in a large sauté pan or pot over medium heat to sauté the tofu and vegetables. Add in the curry paste in step 2 and continue with the instructions.

If You Have More Time

Eggplant is used a lot in Thai curry dishes. You can add 2 cups of chopped eggplant (about 1 medium-size eggplant) or substitute it for the tofu. It takes 5 to 10 minutes longer to simmer, depending on the toughness of the eggplant. Be careful to keep the flame on low; you don't want the coconut milk to boil too much. Other delicious additions are 2 of cups squash, pumpkin, potatoes, or sweet potatoes, if you have a little more time.

QUINOA KITCHARI

Kitchari is considered one of the most healing meals according to the ancient Indian science of ayurveda. It translates as "mixture" and usually refers to a mixture of two grains. On a recent camping trip we discovered an amazing quick and easy kitchari—a one-pot meal that can even be cooked over a fire within thirty minutes. We dubbed it Kalalau Stew or Quinoa Kitchari.

SERVES 4 TO 6

1 cup uncooked quinoa

1 cup dried red lentils, rinsed and drained

5 cups water or stock

1 small yellow onion, chopped

8 whole garlic cloves

¼ cup minced fresh herbs such as cilantro, Italian parsley, and dill

Soy sauce

Sea salt and black pepper

1. Place all ingredients except herbs, soy sauce, salt, and pepper, in a medium-size pot over medium-high heat.
2. Cook until all the liquid is absorbed, about 25 minutes, stirring occasionally. The consistency should be just slightly liquidy. Add more water if necessary as cooking. Add herbs, soy sauce, salt, and pepper to taste.

Variations
- The variations are countless. You can add 1½ cups of your favorite vegetables, chopped small, along with the quinoa. Try carrot, celery, zucchini, cabbage, or asparagus.
- Add 1 teaspoon of fennel seeds and 1 tablespoon of ground cumin or Indian Spice Blend (page 277).
- You may enjoy squeezing some fresh lime juice and drizzling a little toasted sesame oil over individual servings of kitchari.
- Add 1 tablespoon of miso paste and 1 tablespoon of minced fresh ginger or pickled ginger.

JAMAICAN VEGETABLE MEDLEY

Although it would seem that Jamaicans grill a lot, for thirty-minute meals we often prefer broiling for its ease and cleanliness factors. This dish is fabulously accompanied by Baked Plantains (page 186), and Coco Rice (page 195), but some quick quinoa and a side of salad greens are a suitable match as well.

SERVES 4

½ pound extra-firm tofu or tempeh, cut into large cubes (see page 27)

1 tablespoon soy sauce

10 large cremini mushrooms, halved

½ red bell pepper, seeded and chopped large

½ green bell pepper, seeded and chopped large

½ yellow onion, chopped large

10 cherry tomatoes

1 recipe Jerk Sauce (recipe follows)

Jerk Sauce

1 tablespoon ground allspice

1 tablespoon ground cinnamon

1 teaspoon ground nutmeg

1 teaspoon ground cumin

1 teaspoon dried thyme

¼ teaspoon ground cloves

½ teaspoon cayenne, or to taste

1 tablespoon peeled and minced fresh ginger

2 garlic cloves

½ teaspoon molasses

¼ cup agave nectar

2 tablespoons coconut oil

1 tablespoon soy sauce

½ teaspoon cayenne, or to taste

1. Preheat the oven to a high broil. Place the tofu cubes in a baking dish or glass storage container (something with a flat bottom) and cover with the soy sauce by gently mixing well with your hands. Allow them to marinate while preparing the other vegetables. Place all of the other vegetables in a large mixing bowl.

continues

2. Blend all of the sauce ingredients in a food processor or blender for 20 to 30 seconds, or until well combined. Pour over the vegetables and toss until all are coated. Add the tofu, along with the soy sauce, and toss gently. Lay the vegetables out on a baking tray in a single layer. Broil them for 8 to 12 minutes, or until the vegetables are tender on the inside and slightly crispy on the outside. Serve immediately.

Variation

- Try adding spicy peppers to the sauce. Jamaicans are well known for using the hottest peppers around, the habanero and the Scotch bonnet. Yowsers! Go easy!

If You Have More Time

You can also try your hand at skewering. This recipe will make about six kebabs. Arrange each kebab with an assortment of the vegetables, then broil as instructed, rotating once.

MOROCCAN COUSCOUS

Commonly referred to as a grain, couscous is actually a pasta processed from semolina flour. A staple food of North African origin, it's used often in stews and is a highlight in Moroccan cuisine. The distinctive flavor of this dish comes from the saffron, the most costly spice and worth every penny.

SERVES 6

¼ teaspoon saffron threads
¾ cup warm water

Couscous
2 cups water or vegetable stock
½ teaspoon sea salt
2 tablespoons minced fresh Italian parsley
2 teaspoons minced fresh mint
1½ cups uncooked couscous

Veggie Medley
1½ tablespoons olive oil
1¼ cups chopped yellow onion
4 garlic cloves, pressed or minced
3 shiitake mushrooms, sliced
4 tomatoes, chopped (3 cups)
3 tablespoons orange juice
1 (14-ounce) can garbanzos, drained or 1½ cups cooked
¼ cup raisins
½ cup chopped (jarred or canned) artichoke hearts
2 teaspoons curry powder
1 teaspoon ground cinnamon
3 tablespoons minced fresh Italian parsley
1 tablespoon minced fresh mint
½ teaspoon sea salt, or to taste
Black pepper

1. Add the saffron to the warm water in a small cup.
2. To prepare the couscous, bring 2 cups of water and salt to a boil. Place the parsley and mint in a large bowl. Add the boiled water and couscous, and gently mix

continues

215

well. Cover the bowl with a dish towel. When the liquid is absorbed, about 10 minutes, fluff with a fork.

3. Pour the oil into a large pot over medium-high heat. Add the onion and garlic, and cook for 2 minutes, stirring frequently. Add the mushrooms and cook for 1 minute, stirring frequently. Add the tomatoes, orange juice, and garbanzos, and cook for 5 minutes, stirring occasionally. Add the raisins, artichoke hearts, curry powder, and cinnamon, and cook for 10 minutes, stirring occasionally. Add the saffron, the saffron soak water, parsley, mint, salt, and pepper, and mix well. Serve on a bed of couscous.

Variations

- Add 8 ounces of tempeh, or 1 pound of extra-firm tofu, cubed. You can also marinate and roast them before adding (see page 28).
- Replace the tomatoes with two 15-ounce cans of fire-roasted tomatoes or grill them yourself (see page 28).

FAJITAS BONITAS

This dish can be made regularly because it is so simple and yet impressive. We love the flavor and meatiness of the mushroom here, but the recipe also works well with tofu or tempeh instead of the Portobello. Taking the time to serve with rice and beans would make the meal even more traditional. Salsa (page 82), Vegan Sour Cream (page 289), and sliced avocado or Guacamole (page 88) also go well with fajitas.

SERVES 4 TO 6

6 whole-grain flour tortillas

2 tablespoons olive oil

2 large garlic cloves, pressed or minced

1 yellow onion, cut into half-moon slices

1 red bell pepper, seeded and cut into ½-inch strips

1 green bell pepper, seeded and cut into ½-inch strips

2 Portobello mushrooms, cut into ½-inch strips (about 8 ounces)

1 teaspoon seeded and minced jalapeño, or to taste (optional)

½ cup corn, either frozen or fresh off the cob (optional)

2 teaspoons ground cumin

1 teaspoon chile powder

¼ teaspoon cayenne, or to taste

1 teaspoon sea salt, or to taste

½ teaspoon black pepper, or to taste

1 tablespoon soy sauce

2 cups thinly sliced lettuce (about 4 ounces)

1 cup cubed and seeded tomato

1. Preheat the oven to 200°F. Place the tortillas on a baking tray or a plate and cover them with a moist towel to warm them up without drying them out. Let them heat up gently while you make the rest of the meal.
2. Using a large skillet or wok, sauté the olive oil, garlic, onion, red and green bell peppers, mushrooms, and jalapeño, if using, over medium heat for about 5 minutes, or until the peppers are bright and soft, stirring occasionally. Add the corn, if using, cumin, chile powder, cayenne, salt, pepper, and soy sauce, and cook for 5 minutes more, or until all veggies are cooked through.
3. Remove the tortillas from the oven. Serve the sautéed vegetables, lettuce, and tomatoes in separate bowls along with the warm tortillas still under the towel, and let everyone make his or her own.

continues

Variations

- Add 8 ounces of extra-firm tofu or tempeh, cut in strips, to the recipe after the onions in step 2. You can try roasting them for extra flavor (see page 28), in which case you can toss them in at the end or serve on the side as an optional ingredient.
- Substitute 8 ounces of seitan for the Portobello mushrooms and add to the recipe after the onions in step 2.
- If you have more time, serve the fajitas with the Taco Filling (page 228).

LIVE MACADAMIA NUT–RICOTTA VEGGIE TOWERS

You can serve this simplified version of a live lasagne as a light dinner with a side of salad greens or Rainbow Kale Salad (page 138). If you have more time, serve with Pesto (page 246). The ricotta is very versatile—it can be used as a spread on sandwiches or mixed with pasta. Also try the ricotta as a soy-free replacement to the tofu ricotta used in the Zucchini Roll-Ups (page 295).

SERVES 4

1 recipe Live Shoyu Marinade (recipe follows)

1 large zucchini, sliced thinly into rounds

1 recipe Macadamia Ricotta (recipe follows)

2 large tomatoes, cut into ½-inch slices (at least 8 slices)
(large beefsteak tomatoes work wonderfully)

Black and white sesame seeds (optional)

Diced red bell pepper (optional)

Live Shoyu Marinade

1 tablespoon Nama Shoyu

1 teaspoon agave nectar

1 tablespoon water

1 teaspoon raw apple cider vinegar

1 teaspoon freshly squeezed lemon juice

1 tablespoon minced fresh herbs

Macadamia Ricotta

2 cups macadamia nuts

1–1¼ cups water

1 tablespoon freshly squeezed lemon juice

1½ teaspoons raw apple cider vinegar

1 garlic clove

¼ cup minced fresh basil, tightly packed

3 tablespoons nutritional yeast

½ teaspoon sea salt, or to taste

continues

1. Place all of the marinade ingredients in a shallow dish and whisk well. Add the sliced zucchini and allow to marinate while preparing the remainder of the dish.
2. Place all the Macadamia Ricotta ingredients in a food processor and process until smooth. The amount of water used will depend on the strength of the processor. You are looking for a texture that is smooth but not watery.
3. To create the towers, place a slice of tomato on each plate. Spread 1 to 2 tablespoons of the macadamia ricotta over the tomato. Top with two slices of zucchini. Follow with another slice of tomato. Top with another 1 to 2 tablespoons of the macadamia ricotta and another layer of zucchini. Garnish with a sprinkle of black and white sesame seeds and some diced red bell pepper.

Variations
- Replace the ricotta with cashew cheese (see page 291).
- Replace the zucchini with turnips or cucumbers.
- Another way you can present this dish is to reuse an 8-ounce plastic container as a mold to form individual lasagnes. For this, slice tomatoes as thinly as possible. Create a tomato layer, top with cheese, then a zucchini layer, and repeat. When ready to eat, flip the container upside down onto a plate.

PASTA FLORENTINE

Here is another "you won't believe its vegan" experience for all of us pasta lovers. The nutritional yeast gives this creamy dish it's nutty, cheeselike flavor. We recommend brown rice pasta, feel free to use whatever type you like. The smaller, shaped pastas (rotini, rigatoni, or elbows) work best. Try serving along with a large salad such as Arugula (page 134) or Greek (page 144), and whole-grain Garlic Bread (page 192).

SERVES 6

12 ounces uncooked brown rice pasta or other pasta

1½ tablespoons olive oil

1 cup thinly sliced yellow onion

2 tablespoons minced garlic

10 ounces frozen spinach (thawed), or 8 cups fresh spinach, rinsed and drained

1 cup plain soy or rice milk

¼ cup + 2 tablespoons nutritional yeast

3 tablespoons minced fresh basil

2 tablespoons minced fresh Italian parsley

1 teaspoon dried oregano

1 teaspoon sea salt, or to taste

½ teaspoon black pepper, or to taste

½ cup grated vegan mozzarella (optional)

1. Bring a pot of water to a boil over high heat. Add the pasta and cook according to the package instructions, or until the pasta is just tender, 8 to 10 minutes, depending on the variety you use. Drain, rinse well, and place in a large bowl.
2. While the pasta is cooking, add the oil to a large sauté pan over medium-high heat. Add the onion and garlic, and cook for 3 minutes, stirring frequently. Add the spinach and cook for 3 minutes, stirring frequently. Add the soy milk, lower the heat to low, and cook for 5 minutes. Add the remaining ingredients and mix well. Add to the pasta and gently mix well.

Variations
- Add 2 cups of chopped, assorted mixed vegetables, including broccoli, carrots, and zucchini, after adding the onion and garlic.
- Try substituting coconut milk for the soy milk, for a more exotic flare.

continues

Quicker and Easier

For a super simple pasta dish, and a favorite of kids everywhere, add olive oil, nutritional yeast, fresh herbs, sea salt, and fresh ground pepper to taste to your favorite pasta.

Another quick and easy pasta dish is **Pasta Primavera**: Simply add your favorite vegetables such as steamed broccoli, carrots, and cauliflower to your cooked pasta. Add some fresh chopped vegetables, such as celery and red onion, and some minced fresh herbs such as basil and Italian parsley. Toss with Balsamic Dressing (page 144) or your favorite.

ASIAN SHIITAKE TOFU

This is a variation of one of our favorite dishes at a local Chinese restaurant where it is served on a "sizzling platter" shaped like a cow. While perhaps not offering such a classy presentation, you will be quite pleased to serve this over quinoa or basmati rice. Our version leaves out the MSG and uses arrowroot to thicken the sauce. To go all out, serve with Summer Rolls (page 109).

SERVES 4 TO 6

1 tablespoon sesame oil or toasted sesame oil

1 cup chopped yellow onion

4 garlic cloves, pressed or minced

1 tablespoon peeled and minced fresh ginger

1¾ cups water or vegetable stock

1 medium-size bunch broccoli, cut into small florets (2½ cups)

1¼ cups shiitake mushrooms, halved

1 red bell pepper, seeded and julienned

3½ tablespoons soy sauce

1 pound extra-firm tofu, cubed (see page 27)

1 tablespoon mirin (optional)

1 teaspoon Sucanat, organic sugar, or pure maple syrup

1 teaspoon Chinese five-spice powder (optional but recommended)

Crushed red pepper

3 tablespoons arrowroot dissolved in ½ cup cold water

Black sesame seeds

1. Heat a large sauté pan or wok on medium-high heat. Pour in the oil, add the onion, garlic, and ginger, and cook for 3 minutes, stirring frequently. Add the water, broccoli, mushrooms, and bell pepper, and cook for 5 minutes, stirring occasionally.
2. Add the remaining ingredients except the arrowroot mixture and cook for 10 minutes, stirring occasionally. Slowly add the arrowroot mixture, stirring constantly until the sauce thickens. Garnish with black sesame seeds before serving.

Variations
- Replace the broccoli with an equal amount of your favorite vegetables. Try cauliflower, carrots, zucchini, snow peas, bamboo shoots, or water chestnuts.
- You can roast the tofu cubes before adding (see page 28).
- Try replacing the tofu with tempeh.

> ### *Superfoods for Health*
> Shiitake and other mushrooms have been used medicinally in China for thousands of years. They have antioxidants with immunity-strengthening qualities and are reputed to be beneficial for heart health.

MACADAMIA NUT–CRUSTED TOFU

This is the dish to serve when you wish to impress your friends with tofu's delicious possibilities. The crust lends itself to numerous variations. For a thirty-minute meal, serve on a bed of quinoa. You will love it on its own, or if you have more time, serve with Pesto (page 246), Mushroom-Onion Gravy (page 236), or Salsa (page 82). For the ultimate delight, serve with Pan-Seared Oyster Mushrooms (page 178), Gingered Collards (page 177), or Southwest Roasted Asparagus and Corn (page 179).

SERVES 4

1 pound extra-firm tofu

1 tablespoon soy sauce

1 tablespoon coconut oil or your favorite (optional)

1 tablespoon water

Tahini Marinade

2 tablespoons tahini

1 teaspoon soy sauce

½ teaspoon minced garlic (optional)

2 tablespoons water or more, depending on consistency of tahini

Crust

½ cup macadamia nuts

2 tablespoons dried coconut

2 teaspoons blue cornmeal (optional)

¼ teaspoon ground cumin

⅛ teaspoon sea salt

⅛ teaspoon black pepper

1 tablespoon minced fresh cilantro, Italian parsley,
basil, or herb of your choosing

1. Preheat the oven or a toaster oven to 350°F. Slice the tofu into four cutlets. Or try making triangles by slicing the block of tofu diagonally and then slice in half to create four cutlets. Place on a baking dish with soy sauce, coconut oil, if using, and water. Marinate for 5 minutes, flipping periodically.
2. While the tofu is marinating, prepare the tahini marinade by placing the ingredients in a small bowl and whisking well.

3. Place the tofu, along with its marinade, in the oven and roast for 12 minutes. While the tofu is cooking, prepare the crust. Pulse-chop the macadamia nuts in a food processor until they are coarse crumbs. Be careful not to overprocess or they will turn into a paste. Transfer to a bowl with the remaining crust ingredients and mix well.

4. Remove the tofu from the oven and coat the top of the cutlets with tahini marinade, using a spoon. Liberally top the cutlets with the crust mixture and bake for an additional 5 minutes. Serve immediately.

Variations

- So many are possible. You can replace the tofu with tempeh, Portobello mushrooms or small eggplants cut in half.
- For optimal flavor, try toasting the coconut and macadamia nuts (see page 26).
- All or a portion of the macadamia nuts can be replaced with walnuts, pecans, cashews, or pistachio nuts.
- Experiment with your favorite spices and herbs. Try thyme, marjoram, caraway, mustard seeds, or tarragon.

CHIPOTLE CHILE–RUBBED SOUTHWEST TEMPEH

This recipe is a variation of the Spanish Marinated tempeh we serve as part of our best-selling Enchilada Casserole. Chipotle peppers are smoked jalapeños, available dried and in a jar. You can also look for dried chipotle chile powder (we found some incredible powder on our last trip to Santa Fe). Serve with Vegan Sour Cream (page 289) on a bed of quinoa or rice, as part of Mexican fiesta night, or use as a filling for burritos (see page 74).

SERVES 6

3 chipotle peppers, seeded

3 tablespoons olive oil

1 cup water

2 limes, juiced

4 garlic cloves, pressed or minced

3 tablespoons soy sauce

1 (6-ounce) can tomato paste (optional but recommended)

1 pound tempeh

2 teaspoons chile powder, chipotle if possible

1 teaspoon ground cumin

¼ teaspoon ground cinnamon

Pinch of cayenne

1 small yellow onion, sliced

2 large tomatoes, sliced

3 tablespoons minced fresh cilantro

1. Preheat the oven to 425°F. If using dried chipotle peppers, soak in warm water for 10 minutes. In a large casserole dish, combine the olive oil, water, lime juice, garlic, soy sauce, and tomato paste, if using, and mix well.
2. Slice the tempeh into thin cutlets and place in the mixture. Allow to marinate for 5 minutes, flipping occasionally. Combine the chile powder, cumin, cinnamon, and cayenne in a small bowl, and sprinkle it over the cutlets, rubbing it in evenly to coat.
3. Place the onion, tomatoes, and chipotles on top of the tempeh and bake for 15 to 18 minutes. Remove from oven, top with cilantro and serve warm.

Variations

- Replace the tempeh with tofu cutlets, Portobello mushrooms, or eggplant cut into ¾-inch rounds.
- If you don't have access to chipotle chiles, replace with 2 bell peppers, seeded and chopped.

Superfoods for Health

Cilantro, also called Chinese parsley and coriander, is one of the world's most ancient herbs, with written records dating back to 1500 BC. A staple of Indian, Asian, Southwestern, Mexican, Caribbean, and North African cuisine, it has a long history of medicinal use and is currently being studied for its cholesterol-lowering effects.

TACO NITE

Taco night is always a happy night in our house. We enjoy creating unique fillings for friends and relatives but it is just as fun to keep it simple. We don't often use cheese substitutes, but we include it here for transitioners. And if you were inspired by our encouragement to precook your own beans we offer a simple "refried" bean recipe at the end as well.

SERVES 4 TO 6

12 taco shells or soft corn tortillas

8 ounces tempeh

1 cup diced yellow onion

2 tablespoons soy sauce

⅛ teaspoon celery seeds

2 teaspoons chile powder

1 tablespoon ground cumin

½ teaspoon cayenne

Black pepper

1 (15-ounce) can refried beans, traditional or black beans

½ head green or red leaf lettuce, chopped into strips

1 red bell pepper, seeded and diced

2 medium-size tomatoes, chopped

½ cup diced red onion

½ cup minced fresh cilantro

1–2 cups vegan cheese such as mozzarella or
Monterey Jack, shredded (optional)

1. Heat the taco shells or corn tortillas according to the package instructions.
2. Use your hands to crumble the tempeh into small pieces. Place in a pot or sauté pan and cook over medium heat with the onions, soy sauce, celery seeds, chile powder, cumin, cayenne, and black pepper for 6 to 8 minutes, or until the onions are soft and the tempeh looks cooked, stirring occasionally. Add a small amount of water if necessary, to keep the tempeh from sticking.
3. In a separate pan, heat the refried beans over medium-low heat for 6 to 8 minutes, or until hot, stirring occasionally.
4. Meanwhile, prepare the lettuce, bell pepper, tomatoes, red onion, cilantro, and vegan cheese as indicated. Put everything in separate bowls, including the tempeh and beans when they are finished cooking. Serve immediately.

QUICKIE HOMEMADE REFRIED BEANS

Although canned beans certainly do the trick, using home-cooked beans is the best way to ensure quality and freshness. Less packaging is the eco-friendly way to go as well. (See pages 25–26 for bean soaking and cooking times)

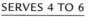

SERVES 4 TO 6

2 cups cooked pinto or black beans

2 tablespoons soy sauce

2 tablespoons olive oil

1–2 garlic cloves (optional)

¼ cup diced veggies, such as onion or red or green bell pepper (optional)

1 tablespoon minced fresh cilantro

1. If the beans are cold, you may want to heat them up first with a little water (about a ½ cup) to soften them. Then, using a food processor (or a really good fork), blend the beans, soy sauce, olive oil, and garlic, if using, until smooth. Some chunks are okay.
2. Place in a bowl and mix in the diced veggies, if using, and the cilantro. Heat if desired.

Tips and Tricks

Because taco shells are a corn product, we highly recommend buying organic if you can find them. Also, look for Eden brand canned beans; they are a high-quality brand.

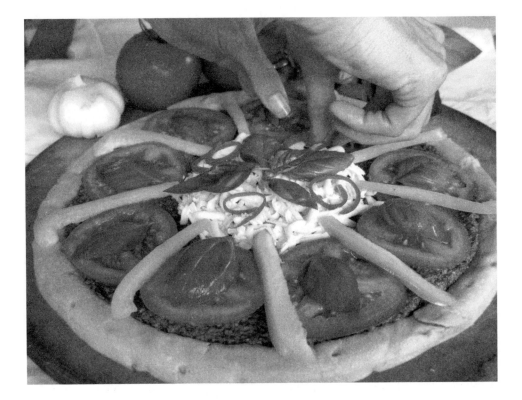

Guilt-Free Comfort Food— Healthy Translations of Old Standbys

J ust what is a comfort food? We all have our favorites, but it seems like the one thing they have in common is that they are often the kinds of foods we are told to avoid or minimize. If it's deep-fried, covered in cheese, and/or made from potatoes, you can be sure that *we* want to eat it, and *they* tell us we shouldn't. Where does that leave a heartbroken, indulgent, football fan with a cold on a rainy day during playoffs?

Chapter 11, that's where. We all feel the need now and then for good ol' fashioned mashed potatoes, nachos, or enchiladas. Even vegans want a burger or some mac & cheese once in a while. Valuing your health and caring about what you eat doesn't make the desire for pizza just evaporate into thin air. Sometimes a salad just isn't going to cut it.

Transitioning to a healthful lifestyle can be a long journey, and we encourage all novice vegans to be patient and gentle with themselves. Incorporating comfort foods that are homemade with healthy, whole-food ingredients is a good step in a worthy direction. That's what inspires us to share these recipes. The fact that they are quick and easy to prepare without compromising on flavor is an added bonus!

CHEESY BROCCOLI

Cheese is usually the last thing a vegetarian gives up before transitioning to veganism. Something about the rich, melty nature of dairy cheese distracts us from focusing on any of its negative aspects. This widespread affection makes creating cheesy dishes a vegan chef's noblest undertaking. We hope you find delight in this dairy-free, cholesterol-free, lower-fat version of a family gathering favorite. You may also use this cheese sauce with many other dishes that call for premade vegan cheese, such as Burritos (page 74), English Muffin Melts (page 97), Quesadillas (page 120), Tacos (page 228), and more.

SERVES 4

1 large bunch broccoli (about 4 cups florets)

Vegan Cheese Sauce
¾ cup nutritional yeast
½ teaspoon sea salt
2 cups soy milk
1 garlic clove, or ½ teaspoon garlic powder
2 tablespoons olive oil
2 tablespoons flour (we use spelt)
½ teaspoon black pepper
¼ teaspoon ground turmeric
1 teaspoon stone-ground or other mustard

1. Steam the broccoli according to the method on page 18 until bright green and tender, about 5 minutes; don't oversteam.
2. Meanwhile make the cheese by blending all of the other ingredients either in a blender or with a whisk (if whisking, you'll need to mince the garlic first).
3. Transfer the mixture to a sauté pan and heat over medium heat for 5 to 10 minutes, or until the mixture thickens.
4. Transfer the broccoli to a serving bowl, drizzle the cheese over the broccoli, and serve.

Variations

- Try adding ½ cup steamed sliced carrots to the broccoli.
- Replace the broccoli with an equal amount of cubed potatoes, or try a fifty-fifty combo. The potatoes may take 3 to 5 minutes longer to steam; put them on the bottom of the steamer basket and steam while preparing the broccoli, if using. Pile the broccoli on top. Steam for 5 minutes more.
- Substitute an equal amount of green beans for the broccoli.

If You Have More Time

For a garnish, thinly slice rings or half rings of yellow onion, sprinkle with salt, and bake at 350°F for a few minutes in a toaster oven until dry and beginning to brown. Spread over the top of the dish before serving.

Superfoods for Health

Beloved broccoli is a member of the cruciferous family of vegetables, along with cauliflower, Brussels sprouts, cabbage, kale, and other dark leafy greens. This superfood dream team is a fantastic source of dietary fiber and is high in calcium, iron, and vitamin C, among many other nutrients.

RAVIN' RAMEN NOODLE SOUP

Latchkey kids and college students across the nation can relate to the simplistic (ahem, addictive) wonder of the ramen craze. It's cheap, filling, and couldn't be easier to make. Of course, even as responsible grown-ups, we still occasionally crave the uncomplicated pleasure of a simple bowl of noodles. And this recipe is all-natural goodness, without the high-sodium, dairy, or processed flavors of packaged ramen.

MAKES 2 LARGE BOWLS OR 4 SMALL BOWLS

6 cups water

4 ounces rice stick or bean thread noodles

¼ cup soy sauce

1 tablespoon dried parsley

2 teaspoons onion powder

2 tablespoons dehydrated onion

½ teaspoon garlic powder

1. Bring the water to a boil in a medium-size pot. Add the noodles and boil for 3 to 4 minutes, or until the noodles soften.
2. Add the soy sauce, parsley, onion powder, dehydrated onion, and garlic powder. Stir, let all of the ingredients sit together on the stove for at least 5 minutes, and serve.

Variations
- You could get really grown-up and add real vegetables to this recipe. We suggest any kind of mushroom, onion, carrot, red bell pepper, bok choy, kale, green onion, and/or fresh herbs. Vegetables should be chopped small or diced, and thrown in with the noodles to give them a few more minutes to warm up. Herbs and green onion can be added at the end before serving.
- Arame, hijiki, or wakame would also enhance this recipe. Add your desired quantity, remembering that the seaweed will approximately double in size after soaking.

ROASTED GARLIC MASHED POTATOES

You will never miss the dairy in this dish that will transport you back to your childhood. We love these potatoes served with Mushroom-Onion Gravy (page 236) or as a side with steamed vegetables and BBQ Tempeh (page 123). We also enjoy how steaming the potatoes takes so much less time, even in large batches.

SERVES 4

2 large russet potatoes, chopped (about 5 cups)
8 large garlic cloves, left whole
1 tablespoon olive oil
¾ cup plain soy or rice milk
Sea salt and black pepper
2 tablespoons vegan butter (optional)

1. Preheat the oven or a toaster oven to 400°F. Place about 2 inches of water and a steamer basket in a medium-size pot and bring to a boil. Chop the potatoes and place them in the steamer basket. Steam them until a knife can pass through easily, about 15 minutes. Drain and place in a large bowl.
2. While the potatoes are steaming, toss the garlic in the oil on a small baking tray and roast in the oven until the cloves are soft and golden brown, about 8 minutes. Place in a blender with the soy milk and blend until smooth. Add to the potatoes.
3. Mash the potatoes and soy milk mixture with a sturdy whisk, potato masher, or hand mixer until the desired consistency is reached. Add the salt and pepper to taste, and vegan butter if using. Serve warm.

Variations
- Try with other potatoes such as Red Bliss, yams, or sweet potatoes.
- Other potatoes may take 5 to 10 minutes longer to steam than the russets. Some people like to combine other veggies with their potatoes, such as carrots, peas, and even steamed broccoli.
- Try adding 2 tablespoons of nutritional yeast for a cheesy flavor.
- Add 2 tablespoons of minced fresh rosemary.
- Spice it up by adding 1 teaspoon of toasted black peppercorns, ground in a spice grinder or blender, or 1 seeded and minced hot chile pepper, such as jalapeño or Thai red chile.

MUSHROOM-ONION GRAVY

One taste of this gravy and you will discover why we included it in our comfort foods chapter. It's rich, satisfying, and has "down home" written all over it. Try with our Biscuits (page 239), Roasted Garlic Mashed Potatoes (page 235) or over tofu or tempeh cutlets (page 27).

MAKES 3 CUPS

¼ cup flour (try whole spelt or white spelt)

¼ cup + 1 tablespoon safflower or olive oil

1 cup thinly sliced yellow onion

1 tablespoon minced garlic

½ cup thinly sliced shiitake mushrooms

2¼ cups water or vegetable stock

¼ cup nutritional yeast

3 tablespoons soy sauce

1 tablespoon minced fresh Italian parsley

¼ teaspoon ground nutmeg (optional)

¼ teaspoon sea salt, or to taste

¼ teaspoon black pepper, or to taste

1. Create a roux by combining the spelt flour and ¼ cup of oil in a small bowl and whisking well.
2. Place the remaining tablespoon of oil in a saucepan over medium-high heat. Add the onion, garlic, and mushrooms, and cook until the onions are translucent, about 5 minutes, stirring frequently. Add the water and bring to a boil. Lower the heat to a simmer and add the nutritional yeast, soy sauce, parsley, and nutmeg if using, stirring frequently.
3. Add the roux and stir constantly until the sauce thickens, about 3 minutes. Add salt and pepper to taste.

Variations

- Replace the parsley with sage or other minced fresh herbs, such as dill or basil.
- You can also create the roux by adding the flour to a pan over high heat and stirring constantly until the flour begins to brown. Stir in the oil until the mixture thickens. This will impart a richer flavor and darker color to your gravy.

TEMPEH-VEGETABLE ENCHILADAS

Enchiladas are normally swimming in cheese. We prefer our enchiladas to swim in fla-vor. Don't be surprised if the sauce seems thin to you; this is normal for enchilada sauce. It needs to cook through everything and it will thicken up by the time they are done. With baking, you may exceed the thirty-minute time frame. If you have more time, try topping them with Vegan Sour Cream (page 289) and Guacamole (page 88), and/or Salsa (page 82).

SERVES 4

1 recipe Enchilada Sauce (recipe follows)
1 recipe Tempeh Vegetable Filling (recipe follows)
8 corn tortillas
1 cup grated vegan cheese such as mozzarella or Cheddar

Enchilada Sauce
2 cups water
1 (6-ounce) can tomato paste
2 garlic cloves
2 teaspoons chile powder
1½ teaspoons ground cumin
1 teaspoon dried thyme
½ teaspoon sea salt
1 tablespoon agave nectar
2 tablespoons soy sauce

Tempeh Vegetable Filling
12 ounces tempeh (usually 1½ packages)
½ yellow onion, diced (about 1 cup)
1 medium-size green bell pepper,
seeded and chopped small (about 1½ cups)
2 garlic cloves, pressed or minced
2 tablespoons soy sauce
½ teaspoon black pepper
2 tablespoons olive oil
¼ cup Enchilada Sauce

continues

1. Preheat the oven to 400°F and lightly oil an 8-inch square casserole dish. Blend all of the sauce ingredients on high speed until silky smooth. Place the sauce in a wide-mouth bowl or container big enough to fit a tortilla.
2. In a separate bowl, use your hands to crumble the tempeh into small pieces. Add all of the other filling ingredients and mix well.
3. To assemble the enchiladas, first dip a tortilla in the sauce and make sure it is covered on both sides. Add about ½ cup of the filling and spread it across the center. Sprinkle with a little bit of the vegan cheese, roll into a tube, and lay in the casserole dish with the seam side down. Repeat with all of the tortillas, stacking them closely next to each other.
4. Pour the remaining sauce evenly over the enchiladas and sprinkle with the remaining cheese. Bake for 15 minutes, or until the cheese is melted.

Variations
- Flavor seekers may soak 1 to 2 dried guajillo chile peppers in warm water for 20 minutes and blend in with the **Enchilada Sauce**.
- For a true Southwest enchilada sauce, heat up the tomato paste with red chiles. Add two to three medium-size red chiles, soaked and seeded, to the sauce ingredients and blend well. You can also use pure ground red chile powder if you can find it.
- Add other vegetables to the **Tempeh Vegetable Filling**, such as red bell pepper, mushrooms, diced olives, or zucchini. Or replace the tempeh with these vegetables for a soy-free version.

If You Have More Time

For a "cheesier" enchilada, use the Nacho Cheese Sauce (page 242) recipe and pour a little into each enchilada as well as on top before baking. Or try with cashew cheese (page 291) for a richer version.

PARSLEY, SAGE, ROSEMARY, AND THYME BISCUITS

When was the last time you made biscuits? This recipe is so easy it could be in "10-Minute Vegan"! Whip them up for a snack, or serve alongside salads or soups, or covered in gravy. You can use whatever herbs and spices you like in these biscuits with no adjustment to the other ingredients.

MAKES 10 BISCUITS

1¾ cups spelt flour or white spelt flour

1 tablespoon baking powder, sifted

½ teaspoon sea salt

1 teaspoon dried parsley

1 teaspoon rubbed sage

1 teaspoon dried rosemary

1 teaspoon dried thyme

½ cup plain soy yogurt

½ cup vegan butter, at room temperature, or safflower oil

1. Preheat the oven to 350°F. Lightly oil a baking tray or cookie sheet, or line it with parchment paper. In a medium-size bowl, whisk together the spelt flour, baking powder, salt, parsley, sage, rosemary, and thyme until evenly combined.
3. In a separate bowl, whisk the yogurt and vegan butter together as much as possible. Add to the dry ingredients and stir with a rubber spatula or wooden spoon. Do not overmix. The dough should be sticky and lumpy.
4. Use a spoon to scoop out ten equal-size biscuits onto the prepared baking tray. Bake for 18 to 20 minutes, or until the biscuits look a little dry on the outside. A testing toothpick may come out with crumbs on it, as long as there is no gooey batter along with it.

PUT THE TEX IN YOUR MEX CHILI

This is a superquick and simple chili that will put the Tex in your Mex. Visit your local ethnic market or ethnic food aisle in the supermarket to experiment with the many varieties of dried chiles available. To enhance the flavor, if you have time, cook at lower temperatures for longer periods of time. Serve with Vegan Sour Cream (page 289) and Savory Toasted Pepitas (page 90).

SERVES 6 TO 8

4 cups water or vegetable stock

1½ tablespoons chile powder

2 teaspoons ground cumin

1 cup yellow onion, chopped small

1 cup sliced celery

4 garlic cloves, pressed or minced

1 (8-ounce) package seitan, chopped

1½ cups chopped tomatoes, or 1 (14.5-ounce) can of fire-roasted tomatoes

1 green bell pepper, seeded and diced

1 jalapeño or other hot pepper, seeded and diced

1 (15-ounce) can pinto beans, drained (1½ cups cooked beans)

1 (15-ounce) can kidney beans, drained (1½ cups cooked beans)

1 (6-ounce) can tomato paste

1 cup fresh or frozen corn (optional)

3 tablespoons soy sauce

3 tablespoons minced fresh cilantro

1½ teaspoons sea salt, or to taste

½ teaspoon black pepper, or to taste

1. Place the water, chile powder, and cumin in a large pot and place over medium-high heat. Begin prepping the onions, celery, garlic, seitan, tomatoes, pepper and jalapeño, and place them in the pot as you go.
2. Lower heat to medium-low; add the beans, tomato paste, and corn, if using; and cook for an additional 10 minutes, or until all of the ingredients are tender, stirring occasionally. Add the soy sauce, cilantro, salt, and pepper. Give it a good stir, and enjoy.

Variations

- For different smoky tastes, try the following: Soak two dried chile peppers of choice in warm water. Remove the seeds, chop, and add along with the other vegetables. Try chipotle, ancho, or guajillo.
- Replace the seitan with 8 ounces of tofu or tempeh, marinated and roasted (see page 28), and crumbled.
- Replace some of the water or stock with tomato juice.
- This is an oil-free dish. If you wish, for added flavor, you may sauté the onions, garlic, and celery in 2 tablespoons of oil for 2 minutes before adding the remaining ingredients.
- For **Chili Dogs**, another popular comfort food, top off a veggie dog with some chili and Nacho Cheese Sauce (page 242).

WE WILL ROCK YOU THREE-LAYERED NACHOS

A football game day favorite, these nachos are a crowd-pleaser. With the tempeh bean dip on the bottom, covered in cheese sauce, and salsa on the side, this dish is not short on flavor or excitement. You may wish to add some diced tomatoes and avocado on top. If you have extra time, go for the tomatillo salsa; otherwise, store-bought salsa does the trick.

SERVES 6

1 recipe Tempeh-Bean Dip (recipe follows)
8 ounces tortilla chips
1 recipe Nacho Cheese Sauce (recipe follows)
1 large tomato, diced (optional)
1 medium-size avocado, diced (optional)
Premade salsa, Tomatillo Salsa (recipe follows), or Salsa (page 82)

Tempeh-Bean Dip
1 (15-ounce) can refried beans (pinto or black)
4 ounces tempeh, crumbled
½ yellow onion, diced
½ red bell pepper, seeded and diced (optional)
½ green bell pepper, seeded and diced (optional)
1 teaspoon soy sauce
½ cup water

Nacho Cheese Sauce
½ cup nutritional yeast
2 tablespoons flour (we use whole spelt flour)
1 teaspoon onion powder
1 teaspoon chile powder (preferably chipotle)
½ teaspoon sea salt
1 cup soy milk
1 teaspoon soy sauce

1. Preheat the oven to 425°F. Place all of the Tempeh-Bean Dip ingredients in a small saucepan over medium heat for 5 minutes, stirring occasionally. Transfer to the bottom of a baking dish or casserole pan. Cover with the tortilla chips.

2. In a sauté pan, whisk all of the Nacho Cheese Sauce ingredients, turn on the heat to medium, and stir for 3 to 4 minutes, or until the mixture begins to thicken (it will continue to thicken as it sits). Drizzle about half of the sauce (or as much as you like) over the tortilla chips and bake for 5 minutes, or until the cheese sauce has hardened and the chips are starting to brown just a little. Transfer the remainder of the cheese sauce to a bowl to serve as a dip with the nachos.

3. Remove the nachos from the oven and sprinkle with the diced tomatoes and avocado, if using. Serve the hot nachos, salsa, and cheese dip immediately.

If You Have More Time

Replace the refried beans with homemade (see page 229).

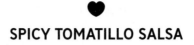

SPICY TOMATILLO SALSA

Luckily our very good friend, Gustavo, clued us in that tomatillos don't need to be roasted to make them into salsa. You don't need to use any lime juice, either, in this raw variation, because the tomatillos are quite tangy enough. Depending on the tomatillos, you may want to use a fine-mesh strainer to strain out some of the water (start with straining just a little and work your way up. This blended type of salsa is more watery than the usual store-bought salsa.)

MAKES 2 CUPS

10–12 tomatillos

2 garlic cloves

1 serrano pepper, seeded, or ½ teaspoon cayenne

¼ cup fresh cilantro, minced

¼ teaspoon ground cumin

½ teaspoon sea salt

Blend all of the ingredients in a blender for 20 to 30 seconds, until a thick liquid consistency is reached.

PESTO PIZZA

Fitting a pizza into a thirty-minute time frame is all about the premade crust. If you have more time, the way to go is to use the Herbed Flatbread (page 192) as the crust. At our restaurant we served a designer pizza du jour, where the chefs came up with creative combinations every day—Thai pizzas, Mexican pizzas, Indian pizzas, you name it. Now it's your turn. Check out some of our suggestions listed below, think out of the box, and have fun.

SERVES 4 TO 6

1 (12-inch) premade pizza crust

1 recipe Pesto (recipe follows)

2 large tomatoes, sliced

1 (10-ounce) package vegan mozzarella (optional)

8 kalamata olives, diced

1 cup seeded and diced bell peppers (assorted colors) (optional)

1. Preheat the oven to 400°F. Place the pizza crust on a baking sheet or pizza stone and place in the oven. Cook for 5 minutes.
2. While the pizza crust is cooking, prepare the pesto according to its recipe. Remove the pizza from the oven and top with the pesto, tomatoes, and cheese, if using. Sprinkle with olives and bell peppers, if using.
3. Return to the oven and bake for an additional 10 minutes. Que bella!

Variations

- Go to town with creating your own designer pizza. Replace the pesto with Tomato Sauce (page 101) and add artichoke hearts and roasted or grilled vegetables (see page 20).
- Replace the pesto with BBQ Sauce (page 123) and top with roasted tofu or tempeh cubes (see page 28).
- Replace the pesto with Spicy Peanut Sauce (page 193) and top with steamed mixed vegetables.

PESTO

MAKES 1 CUP

1½ cups tightly packed fresh basil

¼ cup plus 2 tablespoons pine nuts

½ cup plus 2 tablespoons olive oil

2 tablespoons freshly squeezed lemon juice

2–3 garlic cloves

½ teaspoon sea salt, or to taste

¼ teaspoon black pepper, or to taste

2 teaspoons nutritional yeast (optional)

Pinch of cayenne

Combine all of the ingredients in a food processor or strong blender and blend until smooth.

Variations

- Replace the pine nuts with cashews, macadamia nuts, pecans, or walnuts—use raw or toasted.
- You can add ½ cup more olive oil to create a pesto sauce. Serve with Macadamia Nut-Crusted Tofu (page 224), Pasta Primavera (page 222), Monk Bowl (page 114), or Zucchini Roll-ups (page 295).
- You can replace the oil with an equal amount of avocado, to create a version free of refined oils.
- Add 6 ounces of silken tofu before blending and add soy sauce to taste, for a **Creamy Pesto Sauce**.
- Replace the basil with fresh cilantro.
- Replace half of the basil with mixed fresh herbs, such as parsley and sage.

Quicker and Easier

Skip the pesto and just brush the cooked crust with some olive or flax oil and top with fresh raw veggies, such as tomatoes, red onion, basil, garlic, olives, and/or other favorites. Sprinkle with some salt, freshly ground black pepper, and nutritional yeast, if desired, and you are ready to go.

BURRITO MADNESS

One of our favorite ways to serve this dish is family style, where everyone gets to create his or her own version of the ultimate burrito. Using white basmati rice allows you to fit this in a thirty-minute time frame. If you have more time, you can use a short- or long-grain brown rice (see page 24). The ambitious among you can add our BBQ sauce (page 123) or Nacho Cheese Sauce (page 242) to the standard burrito ingredients listed below.

SERVES 4

1 cup white basmati rice

1½ cups water or vegetable stock

¼ teaspoon sea salt

1 (15-ounce) can refried beans (or homemade, page 229)

1 avocado, seeded and sliced

1 large tomato, chopped

2 tablespoons minced fresh cilantro

¼ cup diced red onion

½ cup grated vegan mozzarella (optional)

4 large whole-grain flour tortillas

Vegan Sour Cream (optional) (page 289)

2 cups chopped lettuce

1. Place the rice and water in a medium-size pot and bring to a boil. Cover and lower the heat to a simmer. Cook for 10 minutes. Turn off the heat and allow to sit for 5 minutes, or until all of the liquid is absorbed, about 5 minutes.
2. While the rice is cooking, place the beans in a small pot over low heat. Cook for 5 minutes, stirring occasionally. You may need to add a small amount of water and watch that it doesn't boil.
3. Warm the tortillas on a griddle or in a large sauté pan. Prep the remaining ingredients as indicated.
4. Build your burrito or serve family style and allow each diner to wrap his or her own. See page 74 for the classic burrito-rolling method.

continues

Variations

- The possibilities are endless here—you're really only limited by your imagination!
- Add tofu or tempeh cubes (see page 27).
- Add grilled vegetables (see page 28).
- Replace the tomatoes with Salsa (page 82) and the avocado with Guacamole (page 88). Replace the refried beans with your beans of choice. Consider the spiced beans used in the Breakfast Burrito (page 74).

Quicker and Easier

A transitional product that makes for a quick and easy comfort food meal is frozen veggie burgers. Amy's is a good brand. They can definitely take the edge off for those craving a burger. First defrost them, then reheat in an oven, toaster oven, grill, or sauté pan. Serve on a whole-grain bun with all the fixings.

There are also veggie dogs on the market. Serve with sauerkraut and mustard on a bun.

MACARONI AND CHEESE

Why is it that macaroni and cheese just keeps putting smiles on kids' (of all ages!) faces? We like this version over the so-called real thing because it is much lower in fat, has no cholesterol, and is so much fresher. Cutting back on processed foods is an honorable achievement for any family . . . and it doesn't have to be labor intensive—nor do you have to sacrifice flavor.

SERVES 4

3 cups uncooked macaroni (12 ounces)

¾ cup nutritional yeast

1 garlic clove, pressed or minced

2 tablespoons vegan butter or olive oil

2 tablespoons unbleached all-purpose flour

½ teaspoon sea salt

½ teaspoon black pepper

½ teaspoon curry powder

1 teaspoon stone-ground mustard

1½ cups soy milk

1. Boil the macaroni according to the package instructions. Drain, rinse, and place in a medium-size casserole dish. Combine all of the other ingredients in a medium-size sauté pan over medium heat, whisking occasionally, until the mixture starts to thicken. It will continue thickening as long as it is exposed to heat; if it gets too thick you may wish to add more soy milk.
2. Pour the cheese mixture over the cooked macaroni and serve immediately.

Variations

- Feel free to add vegetation to your macaroni and cheese. Up to 2 cups of one or a combination of your favorite vegetables, such as broccoli, peas, or carrots, would liven up the mixture. Steam them on the side and mix in with the cheese.

If You Have More Time

Place the completed dish in an 8-inch square casserole dish in a 375°F oven, sprinkle with ¼ to ½ cup of bread crumbs, and cook until the top is crisp, about 15 minutes. To take it up a notch, top with cooked fakin' bacon or Tempeh Bacon (page 57).

HOMEY VEGETABLE STEW WITH DUMPLINGS

This is some old-school stew. We like making dishes like this in 4-quart sauté pans because there is more surface area for direct cooking, which speeds up the process. Although vegetables in stew are generally big and chunky, the smaller you chop, the faster it cooks. If you are a slow chopper, though, you can still do big pieces and it will all work out in the end. The cooking of the dumplings may push this into the forty-minute realm, but your patience will surely be rewarded.

SERVES 4 TO 6

2 tablespoons olive oil

3 garlic cloves, pressed or minced

1 yellow onion, chopped (about 1½ cups)

2 medium-size potatoes, chopped (about 3 cups)

3 carrots, chopped (about 1½ cups)

1½ cups chopped celery

3 cups water or vegetable stock

1 bay leaf

1½ teaspoons dried thyme

¼ teaspoon celery seeds

3 tablespoons soy sauce

¾ teaspoon black pepper

½ teaspoon sea salt

¼ cup + 2 tablespoons spelt flour
(whole or white or even wheat)

Dumplings

¾ cup spelt flour

1 teaspoon baking powder, sifted

¼ teaspoon sea salt

⅓ cup plain soy milk or rice milk

1 tablespoon safflower oil or melted coconut oil

1. Using a large sauté pan or pot, sauté the olive oil, garlic, and onion for 2 minutes over medium heat. Chop the vegetables in the order they are listed and add them as you go to save time, stirring occasionally. Add a little water if necessary, to keep the potatoes from sticking to the pan.

2. When all of the vegetables are in, add 2½ cups of the water and cover. Add the bay leaf, thyme, celery seed, soy sauce, black pepper, and salt, and cover again. Whisk the remaining ½ cup of water with the spelt flour. Add to the pan, cover, and allow it to simmer over medium-low heat while preparing the dumpling batter.
3. In a medium-size bowl, mix the spelt flour, baking powder, and salt. Add the soy milk and safflower oil, and stir. This is a wet, lumpy mixture; do not over-mix. Divide the batter into six dumplings.
4. Give the stew a stir and plop the dumplings on top of the stew. Cover and simmer for 10 to 15 minutes, depending on how moist (or dry) you like your dumplings.

Variations

- Go beyond the obvious stew components by replacing one or more of the suggested ingredients with parsnips, celeriac, pumpkin, cremini mushrooms, or your favorite bean.
- Add some chlorophyll to your stew with your favorite green vegetable. Try curly kale, collard greens, or spinach.
- Add some spices or fresh minced herbs to your dumpling batter. Try rosemary-sage biscuits, garlic-parsley biscuits, or chile pepper–cayenne biscuits.

CHAPTER 12

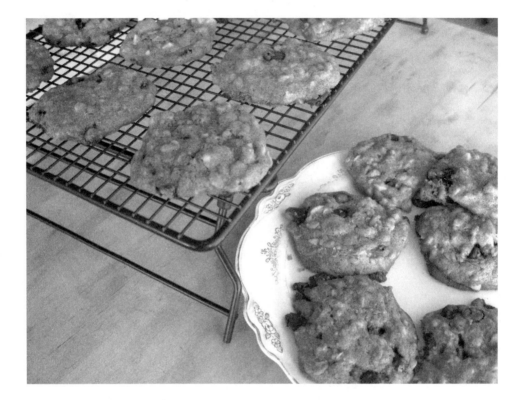

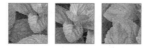

Divine Desserts

Desserts are on the cutting edge of the vegan revolution that is sweeping through the culinary world. These treats have shattered more stereotypes about vegan cuisine than has any other type of food. We get the "I can't believe its vegan" comment more from desserts than from anything else on the menu. Vegan cakes, brownies, puddings, cookies, pies, and parfaits in every permutation imaginable are just as rich, decadent, and satisfying as their dairy- and egg-laden counterparts.

It's a bit tricky to fit all of these culinary delights into a thirty-minute time frame if you count baking time. If you don't count baking or chilling time, pretty much all of the dessert world opens up. For this book, we selected a variety of recipes to share, virtually all of which can be completed from beginning to end within a half hour.

Prepare to discover the sweet mystery of life as you explore the exciting world of vegan indulgence. All of the desserts in *The 30-Minute Vegan* are certified guilt-free and free of refined sugar. We think you will be particularly delighted with our raw offerings, many of which can be a meal unto themselves. The fruit-sweetened Live Pie and the Live Parfait make for a light and filling breakfast.

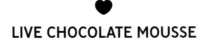

LIVE CHOCOLATE MOUSSE

This is a live version of the "pudding in a cup" we grew up with as a kid. 'Tis so much healthier and just as satisfying. The secret ingredient? Avocado. Yes, we were skeptical at first, too. The key is to use avocados that are neither underripe nor overly ripe, both of which have a superstrong avocado flavor. The pitch-perfect avocado creates a smooth, creamy texture. You can also use this as a filling for a Live Fruit Parfait (page 261) or a layer in a Live Lucious Pie (page 264).

SERVES 4

3 avocados (2 cups mashed)

¼ cup + 3 tablespoons agave nectar, or to taste

1 teaspoon freshly squeezed lemon juice

¼ cup + 2 tablespoons raw cacao powder

3 tablespoons almond butter

Pinch of ground cinnamon

Pinch of ground nutmeg or cardamom

½ teaspoon any flavor extract (optional)
(try mint, cherry, orange, almond, hazelnut, or coffee)

1. Combine all of the ingredients in a food processor or strong blender and process until smooth.
2. If you are using a blender, you may need to add liquid to get the mousse consistency. To keep it live, you can add almond milk (see page 42) or add soy, rice, or coconut milk.

Variations

- For chocolate-orange mousse, add the zest from 1 orange and 3 tablespoons of orange juice.
- Replace the agave nectar with maple syrup or 4 to 6 soaked dates.

Quicker and Easier

Create a heavenly halvah by mixing tahini with agave nectar or maple syrup to taste. Add a pinch of ground cinnamon and cardamom. You can also add some nuts, seeds, or chopped dried fruit as well.

BANANA PUDDING

There are bananas and then there are bananas. Some are supersweet with a strong flavor, others are not. You may wish to have banana extract on hand and adjust the amount of sweetener accordingly. We share two variations here. One version uses silken tofu as the base, the other is raw and uses Crème de la Crème (page 55) as the base. Serve on its own in a parfait glass, or top with fresh fruit. For the next level, top with crumbled Coconut-Lime Banana Bread (page 72), Macadamia Nut–Chocolate Chip Cookies (page 304), Peanut Butter Balls (page 269), or one of the Trail Mixes (page 91).

MAKES 3¼ CUPS

5 small bananas (1½ cups mashed)

1 (12.3-ounce) package Mori-nu firm silken tofu

¼ cup + 2 tablespoons agave nectar, or sweetener of choice to taste

2 teaspoons freshly squeezed lemon juice

1 teaspoon vanilla extract

¼ teaspoon ground cinnamon

1 teaspoon banana extract (optional)

Pinch of ground cardamom (optional)

Combine all of the ingredients in a food processor and process until smooth. You can use a blender instead, in which case you may need to add soy milk, rice milk, or coconut milk to reach the desired creamy consistency, depending on the speed of your blender.

♥

LIVE VERSION

1 recipe Crème de la Crème (page 55)

1 cup mashed banana

2 teaspoons freshly squeezed lemon juice

¼ teaspoon ground cinnamon

Pinch of ground cardamom

2 tablespoons agave nectar, or sweetener of choice to taste

1. Prepare the Crème de la Crème (page 55) in a food processor or a strong blender.
2. Add the remaining ingredients and process until smooth.

Variations

- You can go to town and replace the bananas with blueberries for a blue pudding, strawberries for red (see where we are going with this), and create a layered parfait. Top with a small American flag toothpick and you are all set for the Fourth of July.

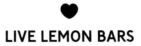

LIVE LEMON BARS

We are huge fans of lemon and lime. Just the smell of citrus can uplift your spirits. These zippy little bars are a powerful pick-me-up. Feel free to decorate the top with bright edible flower petals and dried coconut. Allowing the topping to set pushes this recipe over the thirty-minute mark, but if you don't mind a messy plate, you can enjoy them right away and they will taste just the same.

MAKES EIGHT 2 X 4-INCH BARS

Crust

1½ cups raw buckwheat groats (not kasha)

1 cup pitted dates, packed (preferably Medjool)

2 teaspoons agave nectar

Topping

3 cups sliced banana

2–3 Meyer lemons, zested (2–3 tablespoons zest), or to taste

½ cup coconut oil

1 teaspoon vanilla extract

⅛ teaspoon sea salt

1. Line an 8-inch square baking pan with parchment paper and set aside.
2. In a food processor, blend the buckwheat groats for about 40 seconds, or until they are a fine powder with some whole kernels left. Add the dates and continue to process for another 30 seconds. Add the agave nectar through the top of the machine and process for 20 seconds more. When a piece of the dough is able to be shaped into a tight ball, it is ready. Otherwise, continue to add more agave nectar 1 teaspoon at a time until that stickiness is achieved.
3. Press down the mixture with your hands into the lined baking tray and set aside. Keep some water nearby to dip your fingers in to prevent the dough from sticking.
4. For the topping, process all of the ingredients together in the food processor until a thick creamy pudding consistency is reached. Pour over the crust and refrigerate for at least 20 minutes, or until the topping has set.
5. Use the parchment paper to pull the whole thing out of the pan and place it on a cutting board. Cut in half in one direction and in quarters in the other direction, to make eight bars. Yum!

Variations

- Lime, lemon-lime, orange, and grapefruit are the obvious variations here.
- Other flavor extracts, such as banana, vanilla, or almond, work well.
- Edible floral waters (also called hydrosols) add a taste that is lovely and up-lifting. Try 1 tablespoon of rosewater, orange blossom water, or lavender water. Check the labels, though, some hydrosols are not fit for consumption. Due to the concentrated amounts of plants used to make them, you definitely want to make sure they don't use pesticides.
- Add ½ cup or more of chopped macadamia nuts, cranberries, or dried blueberries.

STRAWBERRY SHORT SHAKE

This knockout of a milk shake was invented to wean a dear friend of ours off her addiction to a devilish little cupcake we sell at our bakery. She used to order them so much we renamed them after her son. Determined to steer her in a healthier direction, this shake was born. Not only does it taste like strawberry shortcake, but it's healthier, faster, and easier to make. If you have access to fresh strawberries, we highly recommend freezing some for just such an occasion. The banana doesn't need to be frozen but it helps with the shake consistency. Adjust the sweetness to your liking.

MAKES TWO 12-OUNCE SERVINGS

1 (10-ounce) bag frozen strawberries

¼ cup cashews or macadamia nuts

1 large frozen banana

1 cup coconut, soy, rice, or almond milk (see page 42)

¼–½ cup agave nectar

2 teaspoons vanilla extract

Pinch of sea salt

1. Blend everything together on high speed until smooth and creamy. This may take a little while (40 to 60 seconds or more).
2. Depending on the strength of your blender, you may need to add a little more coconut milk to get the ingredients to blend.

Variations
- Go all the way and substitute 1 cup of nondairy vanilla ice cream for the banana. You may want to adjust the sweetness, so add the agave last and only as much as you like.
- Substitute your favorite berry for the strawberries. Blueberries, raspberries, black berries, and mixed berries are regularly available in the frozen section.

Quicker and Easier

There are some incredible nondairy ice creams on the market. Check out Coconut Bliss, Soy Delicious, and Rice Dream. These come in countless flavors that are sure to please. Create vegan banana splits and sundaes by adding peanut or almond butter, plus chocolate or carob chips, and topping with Strawberry-Rhubarb Sauce (see page 61) or the Cherry-Vanilla Spritzer (see page 39).

Tips and Tricks

Some blenders come with tampers that you use to move the contents of the blender around while the blender is on. This helps enormously when you are making something thick, such as shakes, smoothies, thicker sauces, or frostings. If your blender doesn't have one and you are comfortable with using a spoon or rubber spatula to stir it up, this would also help. Just be absolutely sure not to touch the spinning blade or it will likely make mincemeat out of your utensil and possibly ruin your food. Or to play it safe, stop blending periodically to stir up the contents.

CHOCOLATE–PEANUT BUTTER SHAKE

This beverage, primarily sweetened with dates, immortalizes the sacred treasure of the chocolate and peanut butter combination. As you experiment with the variations, you will be astounded at the diversity of yummy flavors that are possible. Sheer euphoria awaits!

MAKES FOUR 10-OUNCE SERVINGS

2 frozen bananas

½ cup soaked dates

3 cups rice or soy milk

3 tablespoons unsweetened cocoa powder

½ cup creamy peanut butter

1 tablespoon pure maple syrup

2 teaspoons vanilla extract

Blend all of the ingredients to the high heavens. Behold the wonder.

Variations

- Substitute 1 cup of nondairy ice cream for the frozen bananas, cut the soaked dates back to ¼ cup, and reduce the milk to 2½ cups. We highly recommend vanilla Coconut Bliss.
- For a simple chocolate shake, omit the peanut butter. Add ¼ teaspoon of cinnamon and a pinch of cayenne to make it a Mexican chocolate shake.
- For a chocolate-strawberry shake, omit the peanut butter and add 1 cup (or more) of frozen strawberries (or any berry really).
- Try substituting almond or cashew butter for the peanut butter, adding ½ teaspoon of different flavored extracts, such as orange, coffee, almond, hazelnut, or cherry.
- For a plain peanut butter smoothie, omit the cocoa powder and add ¼ teaspoon of ground cinnamon.

♥
LIVE FRUIT PARFAIT

This dessert will leave you feeling both satisfied and light. Experience it as a snack between meals or even as a light breakfast. Vary the fruits, the cream, and/or the toppings to create your own designer parfait.

SERVES 4

1 recipe Crème de la Crème (page 55)

1 recipe parfait topping (recipe follows)

3 cups assorted berries or your favorite fruit, chopped small (try with bananas, apples, pears, peaches, nectarines, pineapple, mango, or papaya)

Parfait Topping

½ cup walnuts or pecans

3 large pitted dates

2 tablespoons shredded coconut

Pinch of ground cinnamon

Pinch of ground cardamom, nutmeg, or allspice

1. Prepare the Crème de la Crème (see page 55).
2. Prepare the parfait topping by combining all of the ingredients in a food processor and pulse chopping until evenly mixed.
3. Slice or chop the fruit if necessary. (No need to chop those blueberries.)
4. To serve, place 2 tablespoons of the fruit at the bottom of each of four decorative glasses (such as parfait glasses, wineglasses, or brandy glasses). Top with about 2 tablespoons of the crème and 1 tablespoon of parfait topping. Add another layer of fruit, then crème, and finish off with another sprinkle of parfait topping.

Variations
- Add ¼ cup raw cacao to the Crème de la Crème for chocolate crème.
- Replace the walnuts with pecans, macadamia nuts, almonds, or pistachio nuts. Replace the dates with dried apricots or other dried fruit, chopped.
- Replace the parfait topping with your favorite granola.

Quicker and Easier

- ♥ **Stuffed Figs:** Select six fresh or twelve dried figs. Combine ¼ cup of pistachio nuts or hazelnuts, 2 tablespoons of agave nectar, and a pinch of ground cinnamon and cardamom in a food processor and pulse-chop until the nuts are ground. Slice open the top of the figs. Place 1 teaspoon of the filling in the dried figs, or 2 teaspoons in the fresh figs.
- You can also toast the nuts (see page 26).
- Another fig quickie is to split the figs in half and squeeze some lime juice over the top. Ambitious folks can also add some grated ginger.

♥

CHOCOLATE-SESAME BONBONS

As much a conversation piece as they are a unique dessert creation, these bonbons are a lovely alternative to baked goods. The uncommon combination of flavors is the stuff memories are made of. Try bringing these to parties or giving them away as a gift.

MAKES 24 BONBONS

2 cups sesame seeds

½ cup sunflower seeds

1¾ cups shredded coconut

½ cup agave nectar

¼ cup raw almond butter

¼ cup coconut butter

¼ cup raw cacao powder

1 tablespoon vanilla extract

½ teaspoon ground cinnamon

¼ teaspoon sea salt

1. In a medium-size mixing bowl, stir together the sesame seeds, sunflower seeds, and shredded coconut.
2. In a smaller mixing bowl, combine the agave nectar, almond butter, coconut butter, cacao powder, vanilla extract, cinnamon, and salt, and mix well. Add this mixture to the sesame seed mixture and stir until well combined.
3. Using a small scooper or spoon, distribute the batter into about two dozen mini cupcake wrappers. Refrigerate for 30 minutes before appreciating the glory of it all.

Variations
- Use any combination of sesame seeds, black sesame seeds, poppy seeds, and hemp seeds for the 2 cups of sesame seeds called for here.
- Substitute pumpkin seeds for the sunflower seeds or use a combination.
- Toasting the shredded coconut adds another layer of flavor, although if you do this, they will no longer be live bonbons. You could also toast the sesame seeds or bake the bonbons for 10 minutes at 350°F.
- Flavorful coconut butter substitutes are: tahini, almond butter, peanut butter, or 2 tablespoons of coconut oil.
- For a plain vanilla version, omit the cacao powder.
- For a chocolate and vanilla combo, cut the finished vanilla batter in half and add 2 tablespoons of raw cacao powder to one of the halves.
- If using unsweetened cocoa powder in place of the raw cacao powder, use only 3 tablespoons.

Tips and Tricks

You don't need to use a small ice-cream scooper or mini cupcake wrappers as suggested in the recipe. You can use your hands to roll a spoonful of batter into a ball and then flatten the bottom slightly as you lay it on a parchment paper–lined plate or tray to chill. The wrappers do make a fancy presentation, though, and the scooper makes quick work of the project.

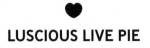

LUSCIOUS LIVE PIE

Fruit sweetened, these treats are high on the list of healthful desserts, with outrageous flavor. You might find yourself having the most fun while decorating these pies with all of the colorful fruits available. The trick to the art of the live pie is to get the filling firm enough so it can slice, although you can get around this by reusing 8-ounce plastic containers (see Tips and Tricks).

MAKES ONE 9-INCH PIE OR THREE 8-OUNCE PIES

Piecrust
1½ cups almonds
1¼ cups pitted Medjool dates
2 tablespoons shredded coconut
¼ teaspoon ground cinnamon
Pinch of ground cardamom, nutmeg, or allspice

Banana Fruit Filling
¼ cup dates
1½ cups mashed banana, not overly ripe
½ cup chopped fruit—strawberries, peaches, blueberries, papaya, mango, or your favorite
2 tablespoons coconut butter or almond butter
1 tablespoon ground flaxseed

1. Prepare the crust. Place the almonds in a food processor and process until just ground. Add the dates, coconut, cinnamon, and cardamom, and process until the dates are broken up and the mixture begins to run up the sides of the processor. You may need to add more dates if you are using a variety that is not as moist as the Medjool.
2. Use your hands to press the crust into a 9-inch pie plate and refrigerate, or press into three lightly oiled 8-ounce plastic containers and freeze. The crust should be about ¼ to ½ inch thick.
3. Prepare the filling by processing all of the ingredients in a food processor until just smooth. Please do not overprocess or the mixture will heat up and take longer to firm up. Transfer to a bowl.

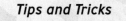

4. If using the 8-ounce containers, remove from the freezer and gently wiggle the crust out of the containers or serve in the container. Pour the filling into the crust(s). Have a blast decorating with your favorite colorful fresh fruits, edible flowers, and shredded coconut. If making a 9-inch pie, refrigerate for an hour or longer to allow the filling to set.

Variations

- For the crust, try using only ¾ cup of almonds, plus ¾ cup of either pecans, walnuts, or macadamia nuts.
- Replace the dates with other dried fruits, such as apricots.
- Replace ½ cup of the crust's dates with raisins. These dried fruits will not stick together with the nuts as well as dates, so add agave nectar—start with 2 tablespoons, and add more as needed to hold things together.
- For a low-fat version, replace the almonds in the crust with raw buckwheat groats.

Tips and Tricks

The advantage of using eight-ounce containers for this recipe is that you do not need to wait for the pie to solidify enough to cut, as they are individual serving sizes. Either serve them right out of the container or, if you are looking for a more elegant presentation, gently pry the crust from the containers. This may take some practice.

If You Have More Time

If you are using the 9-inch piecrust, place the pie in the refrigerator for at least an hour so the filling can solidify enough to slice.

If you are using the 8-ounce containers, keep the crust in the freezer for up to 20 minutes to ensure an easy removal of the crust from the container.

COCONUT MACAROONS

Moist and tropical, this recipe calls for dried coconut because fresh is not so readily available in most places. If you have more time, be sure to go the extra step and top with chocolate. Below you'll find both cooked and raw versions—both are scrumptious, so give them a try.

SERVES 6

1 cup shredded dried coconut

1 cup white spelt flour or whole wheat pastry flour

1 teaspoon baking powder

¼ cup agave nectar

1 teaspoon vanilla extract

¼ cup mashed banana

¼ cup coconut oil

1 teaspoon coconut extract (optional)

1. Preheat the oven to 375°F. Oil a baking sheet. Combine the first three ingredients in a large bowl and mix well. Combine the remaining ingredients in a separate bowl and whisk well. Add the wet to the dry and gently mix well.
2. Using a small scoop, create six mounds from the batter and place them on the prepared baking sheet. Bake until golden brown, about 12 minutes.

If You Have More Time

For chocolate macaroons, melt ¼ cup of vegan dark chocolate chips and 1 teaspoon of coconut oil or safflower oil in a double boiler. After the macaroons have cooled a bit, top them with the melted chocolate. Allow them to sit until the chocolate hardens. If you do not have a double boiler, see page 273 for the Tips and Tricks about the Chocolate Ganache Pie.

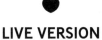

LIVE VERSION

MAKES 10 MACAROONS

1 cup macadamia nuts
1 cup shredded dried coconut
¼ cup agave nectar
¼ cup mashed banana

1. Place the macadamia nuts in a food processor and process until finely ground.
2. Add to a large bowl with the remaining ingredients and mix well. Use a small scoop to form ten macaroons. Refrigerate until ready to enjoy.

Variation

- For a chocolate macaroon, add ¼ cup of raw cacao powder to the mixture.

If You Have More Time

For best results, place the macaroons on a dehydrator tray and dehydrate at 115°F for 10 hours.

You can top these with a chocolate layer as well. Whisk ½ cup of raw cacao powder with 2–3 tablespoons of agave nectar and 3 tablespoons of coconut oil until smooth. Spread over the macaroons and refrigerate until solid, about 20 minutes.

Superfoods for Health

Abundant in tropical climates and a staple food for thousand of years, coconuts are one of our all-time favorite foods. The water from young coconuts is a true elixir, providing vitamins, minerals, and energizing electrolytes. Make sure to use high-quality organic coconut oil. When using dried (desiccated) coconut, use the sugar-free varieties.

FLOURLESS TRAIL MIX COOKIES

Let's not split hairs here, this is a whole different take on cookies. First of all, they're flourless; second, they are loaded with goodies. These cookies are a mystery of baking and they also fit into more categories than just dessert. You can eat these cookies for breakfast or as a bona fide snack. If you omit the chocolate or carob chips, add an equal amount of something else (such as currants, cranberries, or one of the other ingredients).

MAKES TWENTY-FOUR 3-INCH COOKIES

¼ cup pumpkin seeds

¼ cup sunflower seeds

¼ cup almonds

¼ cup cashews

¼ cup carob chips
(preferably grain-sweetened)

¼ cup vegan dark chocolate chips
(preferably grain-sweetened)

2 cups sliced banana

¼ cup pure maple syrup

2 tablespoons safflower oil

1 teaspoon vanilla extract

½ teaspoon baking soda

Pinch of sea salt

¼ cup ground flaxseeds

1 teaspoon raw apple cider vinegar

1. Preheat the oven to 400°F. Process the pumpkin and sunflower seeds in your food processor for about 10 seconds, and transfer to a mixing bowl. Next, pulse-chop the almonds and cashews six or seven times, and add them to the bowl along with the carob and chocolate chips.
2. Process the banana, maple syrup, safflower oil, vanilla, baking soda, and flaxseeds for about 20 seconds while adding the apple cider vinegar through the top of the processor. The mixture should be thick and smooth with a small amount of banana chunks. Add the mixture into the bowl of goodies and stir until well combined.
3. If you aren't using a nonstick cookie sheet or baking tray, you will have to lightly oil the tray or lay down aluminum foil or parchment paper. Use a spoon to scoop out your preferred size of cookie, leaving enough space between them to allow the hot air to circulate and the cookie to spread out (at least 2 inches). It will take at least two trays. Bake them for 15 minutes, or until the bottom edges are starting to brown. Allow them to cool for a few minutes and transfer to a wire rack.

Variations
- Replace any of the goodies you do not like for any of the following in equal measure: macadamia nuts, walnuts, dried fruits like blueberries, cranberries, cherries, pineapple, papaya, apricots, currants, or raisins.

PEANUT BUTTER BALLS

Although we also like old-fashioned peanut butter cookies with the fork marks, we can't help but be a little different. This little treat gives you something more to sink your teeth into. When baked to perfection, the outsides are crisp while the middles are moist. Enjoy them with or without the chocolate chips. And be forewarned, the downside of these is that they disappear quickly!

MAKES 20 TO 24 BALLS

1½ cups peanut butter

¾ cup pure maple syrup

1½ teaspoons raw apple cider vinegar

1 teaspoon vanilla extract

½ cup whole spelt flour

½ teaspoon baking soda

½ cup rolled oats

½ cup vegan dark chocolate chips
(preferably grain-sweetened) (optional)

1. Preheat the oven to 350°F. Whisk together the peanut butter, maple syrup, apple cider vinegar, and vanilla in a bowl. In a separate bowl, sift the spelt flour and baking soda. Stir or whisk well. Add the oats and chocolate chips, if using, and stir well. Combine the wet and dry ingredients and stir again.
2. If you aren't using a nonstick cookie sheet or baking tray, you will have to lightly oil the tray or lay down aluminum foil or parchment paper. Use an ice-cream scooper or spoon to scoop out your preferred amount of batter, forming a ball. Leave enough space in between them to allow the hot air to circulate (at least 2 inches). It will take two trays. Bake them for 8 to 10 minutes, or until they are starting to brown on the bottom.

Variation

- If you prefer a standard cookie shape, follow the same instructions but flatten the balls before baking. The batter will not melt down into a cookie; you must flatten them to the desired size.

ORANGE CREAMSICLE WAFFLES

Belgians created waffles as a dessert. Somewhere along the line, something was lost in the translation and waffles became a breakfast food here in the States. We have combined the nostalgic dreamy flavor of the orange Creamsicle with the fluffy old-world delight of the waffle. Enjoy any time of the day! These waffles cook up the best on nonstick waffle irons. Otherwise, be sure to oil your waffle maker well.

MAKES 6 BELGIAN WAFFLES

2 cups whole or white spelt flour

2 tablespoons baking powder

½ teaspoon sea salt

2 cups soy milk

2 tablespoons melted coconut oil or safflower oil (see Tricks and Tips)

2 tablespoons vanilla extract

2 tablespoons orange zest (zest of about 2 oranges)

Coconut-Maple Syrup

⅔ cup coconut milk

⅔ cup pure maple syrup

2 teaspoons vanilla extract

1 teaspoon orange extract

1. Preheat a waffle maker. Sift the spelt flour, baking powder, and salt, and whisk together.
2. Separately, whisk the soy milk, coconut oil, vanilla, maple syrup, and orange zest. Combine the wet and the dry ingredients and whisk until combined. Cook over medium-low heat or according to your waffle maker's specifications. You may wish to cook for two cooking cycles (if you have the type of waffle iron that beeps when the waffle is ready).
3. Whisk or blend all of the syrup ingredients together. Serve alongside piping hot waffles.

Tips and Tricks

We like to melt the coconut oil by placing it in a mug on top of the waffle iron while it heats up; otherwise, it will harden into chunks in the cold soy milk.

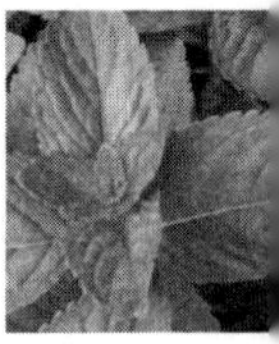

BAKED APPLE CRISP

This is a favorite for kids of all ages. This can just as easily be in the comfort food section. There are over 7,500 varieties of apples, worldwide, many of which are suitable for baking. Try it with different types of apples. Avoid Red Delicious, which are mealy when cooked, and go for Jonagold or Jonathan if you can find them. Serve warm, topped with a vegan ice cream, for the ultimate flavor combination. This will test your thirty-minute capacity as it depends on how fast you can slice those apples.

SERVES 6 TO 8

Apple Layer	Topping
5 medium-size apples, cored and sliced thinly (6 cups) (see Tips and Tricks)	2 cups rolled oats
½ cup apple juice	½ cup flour (white spelt works well)
¾ cup organic brown sugar, or ¾ cup Sucanat plus 1 tablespoon pure maple syrup	½ cup apple juice
	3 tablespoons coconut or safflower oil
½ teaspoon ground cinnamon	¼ cup organic brown sugar, or ¼ cup Sucanat plus 2 teaspoons pure maple syrup
½ teaspoon ground allspice	½ teaspoon ground allspice
¼ teaspoon ground cardamom	¼ teaspoon sea salt
1 tablespoon lemon juice (optional)	¼ teaspoon ground cardamom (optional)
1 tablespoon arrowroot or cornstarch	½ cup walnuts (optional)
	¼ cup vegan butter (optional but will put it over the top)

1. Preheat the oven to 425°F. Place the apples in a large bowl with the remaining apple layer ingredients and mix well. Spread evenly in a 9-inch square casserole dish and bake for 8 to 10 minutes.
2. While the apple layer is baking, combine the topping ingredients in a bowl and mix well. Sprinkle them on top of the apple layer and bake for an additional 15 minutes. The apples should be soft and the topping should be golden brown.

> ## Tips and Tricks
>
> Don't waste too much time regretting that you didn't register for an apple corer. Hold the apple with the bottom on the cutting board and make your first slice just to the right of the center, coming as close as possible to the core without cutting much into it. Lay the flat side down on the board and cut the fruit off all the other sides in the same manner, then proceed with slicing the chunks in strips.

CHOCOLATE GANACHE PIE

This pie is so powerful, magnetic, and distracting you'll want to make sure you have enough people to share it with; otherwise, it may be breakfast. Note that it takes about an hour to chill. This recipe also makes for a good pudding if you don't use a pie shell or if don't want to wait for it to chill. Our sister, Jessyka, happened to find out that this recipe makes rather decadent Fudgsicles if you happen to have Popsicle trays lying around.

SERVES 8

1½ cups vegan dark chocolate chips
(preferably grain-sweetened) (see Tips and Tricks)

½ cup pure maple syrup

1 (12.3-ounce) package Mori-nu firm silken tofu

1 tablespoon vanilla extract

⅛ teaspoon sea salt

1 premade pie shell

1. Melt the chocolate chips by heating them in a double boiler over medium heat (see Tips and Tricks) until the consistency is smooth, lump-free, and creamy, stirring only once or twice.
2. Meanwhile puree the maple syrup, tofu, vanilla, and sea salt in a food processor until smooth. When the chocolate is thoroughly melted (about 20 minutes), add it to the food processor and blend well.
3. Pour the mixture into the pie shell and chill until firm all the way through, about 1 hour.

Tips and Tricks

This dish will come out sweeter if you use the more common semisweet chocolate chips, which contain cane sugar. Sunspire sells a variety that we prefer, which is grain-sweetened, but either one will work—sweeten to your heart's content.

Also, when melting chocolate in a double boiler (which can also be any glass or stainless-steel bowl set on top of a pot with 1 to 2 inches of boiling water in it), be absolutely sure that both the bowl and anything you use to stir the chocolate with are completely dry. A good way to make sure the melting pot or bowl is dry is to start heating it before you put the chips in; this will dry out any moisture. The slightest droplet of water will "seize" the chocolate, leaving it lumpy and devastatingly imperfect looking. But surely do not cry over broken chocolate; everyone still loves to lick it up and your lumpy little pie will still taste divine.

If You Have More Time

Use the Live Piecrust recipe on page 264 for an even more elegant version of this already irresistible pie and top with Strawberry-Rhubarb Sauce (page 61).

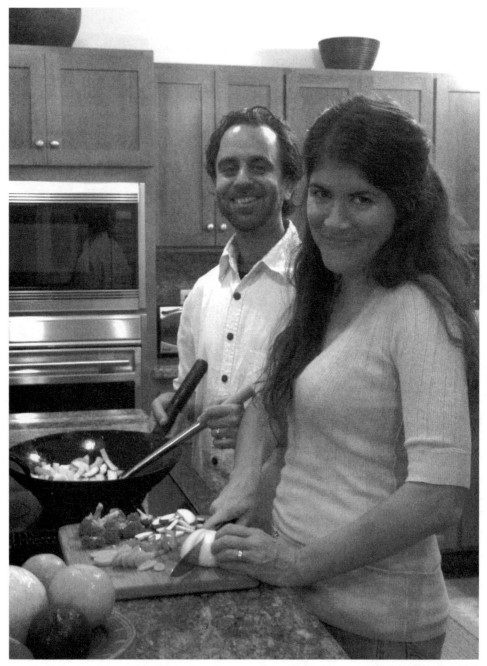

(Photo by Dawn Reinfeld)

CHAPTER 13

Condiments, Infused Oils, and Spreads

Condiments, yummy oils, and spreads are some of the best tricks for helping novice vegans transition fully to a plant-based diet. These are the subtle touches that will transform any dish. They are there for you in those moments when you just need to throw something together or eat something simple without sacrificing satisfaction and flavor.

A simple plate of lettuce is easily jazzed up with a little gomasio, tapenade, or pickled beets. Burn through that ominous mountain of kale with the help of some Roasted Garlic–Chile Oil. Substitute some dairy-free cashew cheese for cream cheese on your next bagel. Use any of the Spice Blend recipes to elevate a dish of steamed vegetables or grains. Having these items on hand allows you creative expression even in a time crunch. You may want to make a couple of these recipes on a day when you have some time to spend in the kitchen. In the days to follow, you'll be glad you did.

Spice Blends

Here we present some of our favorite blends. Make a large batch, store in a tightly lidded spice jar, and use to create an ethnic flare to soups, dressings, salads, and more. Even a simple plate of rice or quinoa will take on new life. The instructions for all are the same: combine in a bowl and mix well. Please be creative and experiment with some of the variations to create your own designer spice blends.

ITALIAN SPICE BLEND

MAKES ½ CUP

3 tablespoons dried basil

2 tablespoons dried marjoram

1 tablespoon dried oregano

2 teaspoons dried thyme

Variations

- Add any or all of the following: 1 tablespoon of dried sage, 1 teaspoon of ground dried rosemary, 1 teaspoon of crushed red pepper flakes, or 1 teaspoon of ground dried fennel.

INDIAN SPICE BLEND

MAKES ½ CUP

3 tablespoons curry powder

2 tablespoons ground cumin

1 tablespoon ground coriander

2 teaspoons powdered turmeric

2 teaspoons powdered ginger

1 teaspoon cayenne

1 teaspoon black pepper

Variations
- Try toasting the cumin and coriander (see page 26).
- Add 1 tablespoon of brown mustard seeds, 1 tablespoon of cumin seeds, 1 teaspoon of fennel seeds, ½ teaspoon of ground cardamom, and ¼ teaspoon ground cloves.

MEXICAN SPICE BLEND

MAKES ½ CUP

¼ cup chile powder

2 tablespoons ground cumin

2 teaspoons dried oregano

2 teaspoons garlic powder

1 teaspoon black pepper

½ teaspoon cayenne

½ teaspoon ground cinnamon

Variations
- Try toasting the cumin and chile powder (page 26).
- Experiment with different types of chile powder if you can get your hands on some.

GOMASIO

Gomasio is a Japanese condiment used frequently in macrobiotic food preparation. We use it often sprinkled on salads, toast, or any number of dishes.

MAKES ½ CUP

½ cup sesame seeds
½ teaspoon sea salt

1. Toast the sesame seeds with the sea salt in a sauté pan over medium heat for 3 to 5 minutes, shaking the pan occasionally to stir them up. Some of the seeds will pop out of the pan. They are done when they begin to brown and smell toasty.
2. Transfer them to a bowl or storage container immediately as they will continue to toast if you leave them in the hot pan. Cool and store in an airtight container. Use within a couple of weeks.

Variations
- Experiment with different flavors by adding 1 tablespoon of ground nori, ½ teaspoon of garlic powder, ½ teaspoon of wasabi powder, ¼ teaspoon of cayenne, or even ½ teaspoon of chile powder.

Superfoods for Health

Sesame seeds are one of the finest sources of plant-based protein and calcium. They are prevalent in Middle Eastern cuisine, especially in the form of tahini, which is made by grinding the sesame seeds into a paste. You can also experiment with making your own sesame milk (see page 42).

CRUNCHY CROUTONS

There is always a use for stale bread because everyone loves croutons. Obviously they are a popular salad ingredient, but fresh ones like these get snacked on all the live-long day.

MAKES 3 CUPS

3 heaping cups bread of choice, cut into ½-inch cubes

1 tablespoon olive oil

1 teaspoon dried parsley

¼ teaspoon garlic powder

¼ teaspoon sea salt

1. Preheat the oven or a toaster oven to 300°F. Place the bread cubes on a baking tray and bake for 10 minutes.
2. Meanwhile, whisk the olive oil, parsley, garlic powder, and salt together in a large bowl. Toss in the bread cubes and stir well to coat.
3. Return to the baking tray and bake for 5 more minutes, or until the croutons are lightly browned. They will continue to harden as they cool. Store in an airtight container at room temperature for up to 4 days.

FRESH THAI CURRY PASTE (RED OR GREEN)

These days, most grocery stores sell some kind of curry paste. Generally it has a thick, uniform consistency with a concentrated flavor from all of the dehydrated ingredients. Due to the freshness of the ingredients in this homemade version, it has a much more watery consistency. Still, you can use it in much the same way as a paste for flavoring dips, spreads, salad dressings, or with our Thai Green Curry recipe on page 210. It will keep in the refrigerator for at least a week. If you don't think you'll use it all by then, you can freeze it.

MAKES 1¼ CUPS

2 stalks lemongrass, cut into ½-inch pieces (about ⅓ cup)

4 kaffir lime leaves

2 tablespoons peeled and minced fresh ginger

4 garlic cloves

½ medium-size yellow onion (about 1 cup)

1 (½-inch) piece fresh turmeric (optional)

2 tablespoons ground coriander

¼ cup soy sauce

3 green or red chiles, seeded

½ teaspoon sea salt

Process all of the ingredients in a food processor or blender for about 30 seconds, or until well pureed. Store in an airtight glass container.

Tips and Tricks

The spiciness of the red and green chiles commonly sold in grocery stores varies significantly. The green tends to be milder than the red. Taste them beforehand to adjust the recipe to your liking. Add some of the seeds if you wish for more heat. You can experiment with any kind of chile you like.

Superfoods for Health

Turmeric is a root of the ginger family. It's a main ingredient in curries and imparts curry powder's yellow color. In its fresh form, it looks like a mini ginger. The Hawaiian word for turmeric is *olena*. Its rich folklore covers thousands of years of use as an antiseptic and treatment for stomach disorders. Science is now affirming some of this ancient wisdom. Its active ingredient, curcumin, is being studied for its effect in treating many modern illnesses.

HOT HOT HOT SAUCE

This is another dish that is not for the faint of heart. We have some hot red Balinese peppers growing in our garden that make a bright red sauce. Try this sauce with whatever hot peppers you have on hand. Serve to spice up all of your dishes. Add a few drops to Pesto (page 246), Enchilada Sauce (page 237), or anything else you want to bump up a few notches. Store in a tightly capped or corked creative glass bottle for a couple of weeks in the refrigerator.

MAKES ½ CUP

5 large chile peppers, or 10 small, seeded if you wish

¼ cup olive oil

1 tablespoon raw apple cider vinegar

3 large garlic cloves

1 tablespoon freshly squeezed lime juice

1–2 tablespoons water

Sea salt

Combine all of the ingredients in a blender and blend until liquefied.

Infused Oils

Infused oils can raise the complexity, and thereby the enjoyment, of the carrier oil by imbuing it with your favorite flavors. Many of the recipes in this book can be enhanced by substituting your own infused oil. We offer three versions here but, as you will see, they are but a few within a limitless list of possibilities. We offer instructions for the three most common methods. One method can be completed in thirty minutes; one method takes little time but has a week or so of infusion time; the third method is done in a jiffy but requires up to three weeks of infusion time. Experimentation will show you the differences.

ROASTED GARLIC–CHILE OIL

MAKES 2 CUPS

2 cups olive oil
1 heaping ¼ cup garlic cloves, roasted (see page 20)
1 hot red chile pepper (optional)

SUN-DRIED TOMATO-BASIL-ROSEMARY OIL

MAKES 2 CUPS

2 cups olive oil
1 cup chiffonaded basil
3 (4-inch) rosemary sprigs
6 thinly sliced sun-dried tomatoes

TOASTED PEPPERCORN OIL

MAKES 2 CUPS

2 cups olive oil
2 tablespoons toasted black peppercorns (page 26)
1 tablespoon lemon zest (optional)

Tips and Tricks

Use thick oils. Thinner oils do not carry the flavor as well. Olive oil doesn't spoil easily; use organic cold-pressed olive oil.

Method #1: Blend all of the ingredients in a blender or food processor. Refrigerate and use within a few weeks. You may or may not wish to strain out the ingredients using a fine-mesh bag or cheesecloth.

Method #2: Heat the olive oil until warm; it isn't necessary that it be hot. Expose the flavor of the added ingredients by chopping or bruising the herbs and breaking open the spices a little bit. Pour the oil over the ingredients, seal, and allow the bottle to sit for a week before using. Refrigerate, and use the oil within a few weeks. Some people feel that this method releases the most flavor.

Method #3: Expose more of the flavor of the added ingredients by chopping or bruising the herbs, and breaking open the spices, and so on. Pour the oil over the ingredients, seal the bottle, and store at room temperature for up to 3 weeks. Refrigerate and use within a few weeks.

Tips to avoid spoilage:
- Sterilize your bottle by boiling it in water for 5 minutes and then leaving it in the sun to dry thoroughly.
- Make sure that everything going into the oil is dry. Water is the main culprit in spoilage. Lay things in the sunshine for at least 5 minutes to evaporate any moisture.
- Heating the oil along with the ingredients may reduce the water content.
- Eliminate any air in the bottle. Use glass bottles, add the flavor ingredients first, and cover completely to the top with oil (even if it is more or less than the recipe). Stir the oil to release any air bubbles within it.
- Label your bottles with the ingredients and date so that you remember how long it has been sitting out and what is inside of it.
- The oil will not prevent anything inside of it from molding; anything over 6 weeks old is likely to spoil. Refrigerate the oil when it is done infusing and only make batches that you will use within 3 to 4 weeks.
- Store all of the oils that contain garlic in the refrigerator when they are done infusing.

continues

Variations

- Infuse coconut oil or agave nectar with vanilla beans and/or cinnamon sticks. Simply place one or two vanilla beans and up to 6 cinnamon sticks into 2 or more cups of coconut oil or agave nectar and allow them to infuse naturally. Coconut oil does go rancid more easily than olive oil, so only infuse what you think you will use within a few weeks. Use in baked goods or dessert sauces, or drizzle over a toasted baguette. The agave nectar could sit either at room temperature or in the refrigerator for weeks on end without spoiling. Use your best judgment. Serve with tea or coffee, in lemonade or other beverages, or in dessert recipes.

Tips and Tricks

Transform raw apple cider vinegar or white wine vinegar into your own homemade **herbal vinegars**. Make sure the herbs are completely dry. Heat the vinegar to warm, do not allow to boil. Fill a mason jar or bottle with the herbs and cover them completely with the warm vinegar. Allow to sit for 1 to 2 months before straining out the herbs and using. Try tarragon, basil, sage, rosemary, or your favorite herb. Citrus zest, cinnamon sticks, and peppercorns are but a few other possible flavors to include.

PICKLED BEETS

Beets frequently don't get used quickly enough in our house, so this is a nifty little trick for keeping them around longer (although the beets are so tasty, you may find them disappearing quickly!).

SERVES 8

4 medium-size beets

¼ cup raw apple cider vinegar

1 tablespoon agave nectar

1 tablespoon olive oil

½ teaspoon balsamic vinegar

1. Peel the beets, slice them in half, and cut each half into ⅛- to ¼-inch slices. Boil in 1 cup of water over high heat, covered, for 5 to 8 minutes, or until you can easily pass a fork through the thickest slices. Strain and return to the pot.
2. Meanwhile, whisk together the apple cider vinegar, agave, olive oil, and balsamic vinegar in another bowl and add to the beets, simmering for 5 minutes. Cool before refrigerating in an airtight container.

TAPENADE

This is the ultimate quick and easy spread that no home should be without, the dish you want to whip up superfast if guests arrive unannounced. Try it with different types of olives, experiment with different herbs, and you will be amazed at how unique each variation is. Serve with bread, cucumber slices, or Crostini (see page 182).

MAKES ¾ CUP

1 cup olives, kalamata or your favorite
2 teaspoons minced fresh garlic
2 teaspoons freshly squeezed lemon juice
½ teaspoon capers (optional)
½ teaspoon dried thyme
1 teaspoon minced fresh rosemary
1 teaspoon minced fresh basil
⅓ teaspoon black pepper
2 teaspoons nutritional yeast (optional)

1. Gently pulse-chop all of the ingredients in a food processor. Be sure not to over-process or the tapenade will be pasty. You can also mince the olives thoroughly with a knife and combine with the other ingredients in a bowl and mix well.
2. If you have time to let it sit in the refrigerator for 20 minutes or longer, the flavor improves with age.

Variations
- For a unique twist on this, dice three shiitake mushrooms. Sauté them with 1 tablespoon of oil in a small pan until golden brown, stirring frequently. Add to above, along with 2 tablespoons of diced red bell pepper, after the pulse-chopping.
- Spice it up by adding one chile pepper, seeded and diced.

CHUTNEY DU JOUR

Chutney is India's answer to salsa. It's typically made from fruit, with sour elements and a bit of spiciness. This is a versatile formula for successful chutney. We love making ours with mangoes. See the variations for other suggestions. Serve with all of your Indian feasts and with Jamaican Vegetable Medley (see page 213). Serve with tortilla chips as a unique dipping experience.

MAKES APPROXIMATELY 3 CUPS

2½ cups firm and ripe mango, peeled and chopped
(see Tips and Tricks, page 54)

½ cup chopped dried apricots

2 tablespoons raw apple cider vinegar

1 tablespoon pure maple syrup, agave nectar,
Sucanat, or organic sugar

½ cup diced yellow onion

1 tablespoon peeled and minced ginger

1½ teaspoons seeded and minced jalapeño

1 tablespoon minced fresh mint

¼ teaspoon ground allspice

Pinch of ground cinnamon

Pinch of ground cardamom

Pinch of crushed red pepper

Zest of 1 small lime

⅛–¼ teaspoon sea salt, or to taste

1. Place all of the ingredients in a pot over low heat and cook for about 10 minutes, stirring frequently.
2. You can also enjoy this as a raw dish by placing all of the ingredients in a bowl and mixing well.

Variations
- Replace the mango with papayas, green tomatoes, pineapple, or bananas.
- Replace the apricots with dates or other dried fruits.

VEGAN MAYONNAISE

You can use premade vegan mayo (such as Vegenaise) or you can make your own. This homemade mayo is suitable for all recipes in this book that call for mayonnaise. For best results, store in an airtight glass container in the refrigerator and use within a week.

MAKES 2¼ CUPS

1½ cups safflower oil

¾ cup soy milk

½ teaspoon Dijon mustard

1 teaspoon agave nectar (optional)

¾ teaspoon sea salt, or to taste

1½ teaspoons freshly squeezed lemon juice

1. Combine all of the ingredients except the lemon juice in a blender and blend until smooth.
2. Slowly add the lemon juice through the top while blending, until the mixture thickens.

VEGAN SOUR CREAM

Here are two variations for your sour cream enjoyment. The first version has a more authentic sour cream taste. The live version is macadamia or cashew based. Try serving with, among many other dishes, Burritos (page 247), Tacos (page 228), or Seasoned Spuds (page 68).

MAKES 1 CUP

1 cup Vegenaise or Vegan Mayonnaise (page 288) or other vegan mayo
1–2 tablespoons freshly squeezed lemon juice
Pinch of fresh or dried dill (optional)

Combine all of the ingredients in a large bowl and whisk well. Store in an airtight container in the refrigerator for 5 to 7 days.

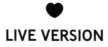

LIVE VERSION

MAKES 1⅔ CUPS

1 cup macadamia nuts or cashews
½ cup water
3 tablespoons freshly squeezed lemon juice
¾ teaspoon sea salt, or to taste

Combine all of the ingredients in a strong blender and blend until smooth. Store in a glass jar in the refrigerator for up to 4 days.

GARLIC-HERB AIOLI

Traditional aioli (pronounced a-o-lee) is an emulsion of garlic and olive oil, sometimes employing eggs for their bonding properties. This simple recipe uses vegan mayonnaise as a base. Feel free to play with other ingredients. Serve aioli as a spread on sandwiches and wraps, alongside Seasoned Spuds (page 68), or as a versatile dip.

MAKES 1 CUP

1 cup Vegenaise, Vegan Mayonnaise (page 288), or other vegan mayo

1–2 garlic cloves, pressed or minced

1 tablespoon minced fresh Italian parsley

¾ teaspoon minced fresh rosemary

½ teaspoon fresh thyme

Stir together all of the ingredients and store in an airtight container in the refrigerator for up to 1 week.

Variation

- For chipotle aioli, add 1 to 2 chipotle chiles, soaked until soft, then seeded and minced.

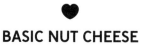

BASIC NUT CHEESE

This simple recipe forms the base of many nut and seed cheeses. Some of our favorites include cashew, macadamia, and pine nut cheeses. For best results, follow the soaking chart on page 43 before blending. Experiment with different combinations for different flavors. Use these nut cheeses as dips for crudités and crackers, or as spreads for bagels or toast, or in wraps and Live Nori Rolls (page 111). The simplest cheese consists of the nut or seed and water. The ingredients we list here will add a more "cheesy" flavor.

MAKES 2 CUPS

2 cups nuts or seeds

1¼–1½ cups water—depending on blender strength

3 tablespoons nutritional yeast

2 teaspoons freshly squeezed lemon juice

1½ teaspoons raw apple cider vinegar

1½ tablespoons or more minced fresh herbs

½ teaspoon minced garlic

Sea salt or Nama shoyu

1. Rinse and drain the nuts or seeds. Place them in a food processor or strong blender and blend, slowly adding the water, until a creamy texture is reached.
2. Transfer to a bowl with the remaining ingredients and mix well.

Variations
- Experiment with different combinations of nuts and seeds. Try:
  1½ cups macadamia nuts or pine nuts and ½ cup hemp seeds
  1 cup macadamia nuts and 1 cup pine nuts
  1 cup cashews, ½ cup pine nuts, and ½ cup sunflower seeds
- Experiment with your favorite herbs. Vary the type and quantity.

If You Have More Time

To add additional tang to the cheese, blend the nuts or seeds and water until creamy. Place in a glass jar (we have a 1-gallon jar for this purpose) and cover with plastic wrap secured with a rubber band, but not a lid. Allow to sit at room temperature in a dark place overnight. Cheese should bubble up as the culturing process occurs. Beneficial bacteria, good for intestinal flora, are created by this process. In the following morning, you can simply add sea salt to taste or any of the ingredients listed in the recipe. The flavor will be tangy and cheesy, which is normal.

For almonds, it is best to blanch them to remove the skins before using in a cheese. Soak for 4 to 6 hours and then place in boiling water for 10 seconds before placing in cold water. The skins pop off easily.

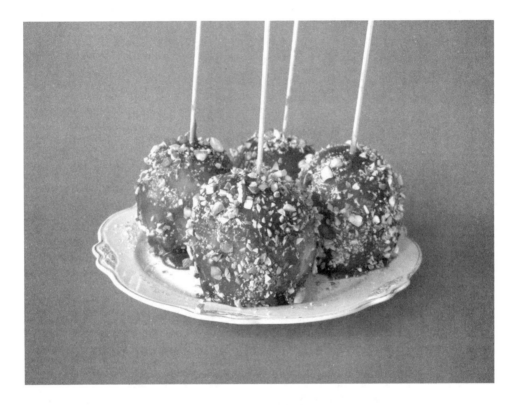

CHAPTER 14

Feasts, Soirees, & Slumber Parties— Quick, Healthy, & Bountiful

Since the beginning of time, humans have been sharing meals, a universal ritual that encompasses the globe. This chapter highlights some of our favorite menu suggestions for a variety of gatherings. Of course, you can vary these menus with any of our *30-Minute Vegan* recipes.

Although each of the recipes can be prepared within thirty minutes, combining the recipes to create a menu will take some planning. Pace yourself. You may wish to prepare some items, or prep some of the main ingredients, the day before the big event. If you are hosting a party, consider doing as much as possible the day before the event, including setting the table and decorating, so you are not rushing at the last minute.

We feature menus for a dinner party, kid's slumber party, BBQ picnic, a live foods soiree, and a holiday feast. Of course, you can also adapt these suggestions for throwing your own themed parties and events. A Mexican fiesta can include Tortilla Soup (page 163), Nachos (page 242) with Guacamole (page 88), and

Enchiladas (page 237). Make an Italian feast out of Insalata Caprese (page 183), Polenta Triangles (page 190) with Pesto (page 246), and Pasta Florentine (page 221). Your India Night can feature Indian Chai Latte (page 40), Red Lentil Dhal (page 167), Tofu Saag (page 209), and simple Coco Rice (page 195). It's fun to decorate with artwork, and play music from different cultures to complement the showcased cuisine. Try fun combinations of recipes in this book for a multiethnic vegan feast extraordinaire!

Celebrate Good Times Dinner Party

Looking for a simple menu that will wow your friends and family? Here is our suggested menu for an unforgettable evening. You can bump it up a notch by replacing the stir-fry with Spinach-Herb Stuffed Portobellos (page 204) or Thai Green Curry (page 210).

Zucchini Roll-Ups (recipe follows)
Salad with Dressing of choice (page 128)
Easy as Pie Stir-Fry (recipe follows)
Coco Rice—with or without the beans (page 195)
Cherry-Vanilla Spritzer (page 39)
Chocolate-Covered Strawberries (recipe follows)

ZUCCHINI ROLL-UPS

Inspired on a romantic gondola trip in Venice (we can dream, can't we?), the vegan "ricotta" made from tofu, tahini, and nutritional yeast is what makes this dish. Be sure to use the extra-firm tofu to keep the consistency ricotta like. Enjoy as is, drizzled with olive oil and freshly ground pepper, or served with Pesto (page 246) or Tomato Sauce (page 101). This dish lends itself to beautiful presentation as an hors d'oeuvre or appetizer.

MAKES APPROXIMATELY 18 ROLL-UPS

2 zucchini

1 pound extra-firm tofu, crumbled

2 tablespoons minced fresh basil

2 tablespoons minced fresh Italian parsley

1 teaspoon minced fresh rosemary

3 tablespoons creamy tahini

2 tablespoons nutritional yeast

½ teaspoon dried thyme

½ teaspoon dried oregano

1 teaspoon sea salt, or to taste

¼ teaspoon black pepper, or to taste

1. Preheat the oven to 400°F and well oil a baking sheet. Slice each zucchini lengthwise into nine or more thin strips (about ⅛ inch side), using either a mandoline (careful of those fingers) or a vegetable peeler.
2. Combine the tofu and the remaining ingredients in a large mixing bowl and mix well. If the tahini is not creamy, you may need to add a bit of olive oil to maintain a creamy consistency. Spread about 2 tablespoons of this mixture along each piece of zucchini and roll it up.
3. Place the rolls on the baking sheet and bake for 10 minutes, then remove from the oven. Serve on a platter or with two to three rolls per individual plate. Refrigerate if you are not serving immediately. The rolls are awesome chilled as well.

Variation
- Replace the zucchini with thinly sliced eggplant.

EASY AS PIE STIR-FRY

This dish boasts a beautiful rainbow of vegetables. Be sure not to over-stir-fry or the veggies will lose their vibrant colors. Slightly crisp vegetables are what you are aiming for here.

SERVES 8

1 tablespoon toasted sesame oil

4 garlic cloves, pressed or minced

¼ cup peeled and minced fresh ginger

1 medium-size yellow onion, sliced into half-moons

1 medium-size red bell pepper, seeded and sliced

1½ cups diagonally sliced carrots

2 small yellow summer squash, sliced into half-moons

2 cups broccoli florets

2 cups thinly sliced red cabbage

¼ cup soy sauce

2 tablespoons pure maple syrup

¼ teaspoon cayenne, or to taste (optional)

6 cups thinly sliced bok choy

1. Heat a wok or stockpot over medium heat. Place the oil, garlic, and ginger in the pot and lower the heat to low. Chop and add the onion, red bell pepper, carrots, squash, broccoli, and red cabbage one at a time as you go. (If you are using a wok, you can scoot the cooked veggies up the sides while placing the new vegetable at the bottom to cook.)
2. Add the soy sauce, maple syrup, and cayenne, if using. Turn the heat back up to medium, add the bok choy, and stir for 2 to 3 minutes, until the bok choy softens. Remove from the heat and serve.

Variations
- Toast ¼ cup of sesame seeds (page 26) and stir in at the end.
- Add 1 teaspoon of Chinese five-spice powder, or to taste.
- Add roasted tofu or tempeh cubes (see page 28).

CHOCOLATE-COVERED STRAWBERRIES

Look for the plump and juicy berries with a deep red color. Covered in chocolate, they are irresistible. You won't be surprised when your guests are feeding these to each other!

MAKES 16 STRAWBERRIES

1 pound strawberries
1 (10-ounce) bag vegan dark chocolate chips (about 2 cups)

1. Melt the chocolate chips according to the method on page 273. Meanwhile, rinse and pat dry the strawberries.
2. Dip each strawberry in the melted chocolate and shake it around so that the chocolate thoroughly coats all of the tiny indentations. Remove, give it a swirl, and place on a parchment paper–lined tray. Refrigerate until the chocolate hardens, about 15 minutes.

Variations
- Other fruits work well here, too. Try this with banana slices. Also try with whole bananas: cover in chopped toasted almonds or pecans (see page 26) and freeze if desired.

The Ultimate Kids' Slumber Party

Feeding a group of kids can have its challenges. This menu is great for younger kids who tend to gravitate more toward simpler transitional foods and rely on old standbys (see the Phoney Baloney Sandwiches). If your young guests are a little more adventurous, consider introducing them to ethnic foods. Mexican is a good place to start. Try Quesadillas (page 120) and Fajitas (page 217) in place of Finger Sandwiches and Mac N Cheese.

Kids' Finger Sandwiches (recipe follows)
Mac N Cheese (page 249)
Crispy Kale (page 86)
Watermelon Cooler (page 45)
Candy Apples (recipe follows)
Spirulina Popcorn (page 84)

KIDS' FINGER SANDWICHES

These are the simple, classic children's sandwiches. Feel free to try to squeak some vegetables in there as well. It's all about the presentation—for finicky kids, healthy foods presented in a cute way make them more appealing. Having some peanut butter and jelly on standby is a good tactic in case of emergency.

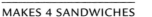

MAKES 4 SANDWICHES

Cucumber Sandwiches

1 medium-size cucumber

Vegenaise or Vegan Mayonnaise (page 288)

4 pieces romaine lettuce

Fresh herbs, if you dare

8 slices whole-grain bread or bread of choice

Phoney Baloney Sandwiches

8–16 slices vegan baloney or
other vegan cold cuts

Vegenaise or Vegan Mayonnaise (page 288),
or substitute favorite salad dressing

4–8 pieces romaine lettuce (optional)

8 slices tomato (optional)

8 slices whole-grain bread or
bread of choice

1. Assemble all of the sandwiches according to the time-honored method. Remove the crusts if necessary.
2. Cut into cute shapes, such as four simple triangles or squares. Or get even fancier and use different shaped cookie cutters. Stars and hearts are two kids' favorites.

continues

Variation

- You can also use flour tortilla wraps to make roll-ups rather than sandwiches. You may have to use toothpicks to hold the pieces together. (If you use something like peanut butter, you have the stickiness factor helping to keep it together, otherwise they may unroll when you cut them.) Lay all of the ingredients across the whole wrap, avoiding the edge by a half inch. Roll it up and insert four frilly toothpicks, evenly spaced. Cut and arrange on a plate. Let the age of your guests determine whether they are ready to deal with the toothpicks.

Tips and Tricks

Admittedly, thinner sandwiches take better to the cookie-cutter method. Also good to know is that the small cookie cutters don't work so well because the details get lost when cutting into such a bulky medium. So go for larger cutters (although you may only get one to two cuts per sandwich, you can still be creative with the trimmed pieces) with less detail (i.e., avoid snowmen, witches). Display them on colorful plates with some small toy figurines on them. Most important, have fun!

CANDY APPLES

You can serve these the old-fashioned way, like a huge lollipop, or as sliced apples covered in caramel sauce. The latter method ensures a greater caramel-to-apple ratio. Traditionally caramel is made by heating white sugar, butter, and heavy cream to high temperatures. We like to think we've taken it a couple steps toward healthy with this version.

MAKES 4 CANDIED APPLES

4 Pink Lady, Gala, or other apples

1 cup Silk creamer or soy milk

½ cup organic brown sugar

1 teaspoon vanilla extract

1 tablespoon arrowroot

¼ cup water

2 tablespoons vegan butter

2 tablespoons pure maple syrup

½ teaspoon ground cinnamon

Pinch of sea salt

1 cup chopped toasted almonds or walnuts (see page 26)

1. It is best that the apples be at room temperature so that condensation doesn't prevent the caramel from sticking. Either slice the apples or insert your desired handle (Popsicle sticks, bamboo skewers, or even forks do the trick) into the bottoms.
2. Whisk the creamer, brown sugar, and vanilla in a medium-size pot over medium heat. Bring the mixture to a boil and simmer for 5 minutes. Whisk the arrowroot and water together and then whisk it into the sauce. Simmer for another 3 minutes, whisking occasionally. Add the vegan butter, maple syrup, cinnamon, and salt. Simmer for 2 more minutes and remove from the heat.
3. Wait a few minutes for the mixture to start thickening and then pour the sauce over either the sliced or whole apples. Sprinkle with the toasted nuts, if using, or roll the whole coated apple in them. Let the whole apples cool in the fridge; the sliced apples can be eaten immediately.

Summertime Fun BBQ Picnic

A tall glass of limeade, corn on the cob, the smell of the grill, and chocolate chip cookies come together to make your day. Whether it's a family reunion, company picnic, beach party, block party, or just a nice little Saturday, this menu wins big smiles. Put a little extra effort in and make Jamaican Skewers (page 214) instead of the Tempeh Sandwich. Try switching out the cookies for Peanut Butter Balls (page 269), Coleslaw (page 140) for the Grilled Vegetable Salad, Chips and Guacamole (page 88) for the Bruschetta.

Bruschetta (page 182)
Grilled Vegetable Salad (recipe follows)
BBQ Tempeh Sandwich (page 123)
Corn on the Cob (page 87)
Lovely Limeade (page 38)
Macadamia Nut–Chocolate Chip Cookies (recipe follows)

GRILLED VEGETABLE SALAD

Whether you enjoy this as a salad or leave the vegetables whole as a side dish, it is light, colorful, bursting with flavor, and a simple joy to create. You can use an outdoor grill or a handy indoor version that fits on the stove with a grill on one side and a griddle on the other. You can also roast the veggies in the oven (see page 20) instead of grilling. Depending on how long it takes for your grill to get up to speed, the preheating may push the recipe beyond the thirty-minute time frame. To avoid this, preheat the grill before you gather the ingredients.

SERVES 4

1 recipe Balsamic Marinade
(recipe follows)

1 large Portobello mushroom

1 large zucchini, cut into ¼-inch slices

1 yellow onion, cut into large slices

1 large red bell pepper, halved and seeded

2 baby bok choy, halved

2 tablespoons minced fresh basil
or Italian parsley

Sea salt and black pepper

Balsamic Marinade

3 tablespoons olive oil

2 tablespoons soy sauce

2 teaspoons balsamic vinegar

1 teaspoon Dijon or
stone-ground mustard

2 teaspoons pure maple syrup

2 teaspoons freshly squeezed lime juice

1 tablespoon water

½ teaspoon minced fresh garlic

1. Preheat a grill. Prepare the marinade by placing all of the ingredients in a shallow dish and whisking well. Place the vegetables in the marinade, coating them well.
2. Grill the vegetables, flipping occasionally with tongs, and cooking until grill marks appear. Remove, chop into 1-inch pieces, and place in a large bowl with the remainder of the marinade and fresh herbs. Add salt and pepper to taste.

Variations
- Try adding pineapple, eggplant, corn on the cob, coconut meat, or baby carrots and grilling with the other vegetables.
- Try serving the grilled vegetable medley over a plate of organic mixed greens. Another pretty presentation would be to lay down two or three romaine leaves, top with the grilled veggies, and drizzle with Vegan Ranch Dressing (page 133).

MACADAMIA NUT–CHOCOLATE CHIP COOKIES

No picnic would be complete without an old-fashioned chocolate chip cookie! Well, maybe it's new-fashioned. One thing we know for sure, if you don't tell anyone they're vegan, people certainly aren't going to guess. Since there are no eggs, this recipe calls for tapioca flour as a binding agent. Tapioca flour is more accessible than you think, if you ask around at the store, but cornstarch can replace it in a pinch (see Tips and Tricks). For the record, these don't bake up as crisp on stoneware.

MAKES TWENTY-FOUR 3-INCH COOKIES

1¾ cups whole spelt flour

¼ cup tapioca flour or other suggested binder

¾ teaspoon baking soda

½ teaspoon sea salt

⅛ teaspoon ground cinnamon

¾ cup rolled oats

1 cup chopped macadamia nuts

1 cup vegan dark chocolate chips (preferably grain-sweetened)

⅔ cup pure maple syrup

⅔ cup safflower oil

2 tablespoons water

1 teaspoon vanilla extract

1. Preheat the oven to 350°F. Sift the spelt flour, tapioca flour, baking soda, salt, and cinnamon through a fine-mesh strainer or sifter. Whisk well and add the oats, macadamia nuts, and chocolate chips, stirring again.
2. In a 2-cup measuring cup, combine the maple syrup, safflower oil, water, and vanilla, and whisk together. Add to the flour mixture and stir well.
3. If you aren't using a nonstick cookie sheet or baking tray, you will have to lightly oil the tray or lay down aluminum foil. Use a spoon to scoop out your preferred size of cookie, leaving enough space in between them to allow the hot air to circulate and the cookie to spread out (at least 2 inches). It will take at least two trays. Bake them for 10 minutes, until the bottom edges start to brown; do not overbake. Allow them to cool for a few minutes and transfer to a wire rack.

Tips and Tricks

Tapioca flour can often be found in the Asian food section of grocery stores and possibly in the baking section as well. You can also find it in health food stores, which are likely to carry it in small bags. Substitutions for tapioca flour are arrowroot powder, cornstarch, or Ener-G Egg Replacer. Arrowroot can be substituted in equal measure. Cornstarch is about twice as strong so, for this recipe, only use 2 tablespoons of cornstarch and add 2 tablespoons of the spelt flour as well. Follow the instructions on the Egg Replacer package for replacing 1 egg. You can also mix 1 tablespoon of ground flaxseeds with 3 tablespoons of water as a replacement for 1 egg.

Live Food Soiree

Whether you feast on living foods regularly or you just want to impress your friends with cutting-edge cuisine, this menu makes quick work for your plan. Starting everyone off with a Supertonic Elixir is your springboard to success. By the time the Live Pie hits the table, you will have a crowd of believers! You can replace the Live Spring Rolls with Rawvioli Provencal (page 180), Un-Stir-Fry with Live Macadamia Nut–Ricotta Veggie Towers (page 219), and the live pie with any of the awesome live desserts in chapter 12.

Supertonic Elixir (recipe follows)
Live Spring Rolls (recipe follows)
Rainbow Kale Salad (page 138)
Live Un-Stir-Fry with Cauliflower Rice (page 198)
Luscious Live Pie (page 264)

SUPERTONIC ELIXIR

This recipe is provided courtesy of Gia Baiocchi, the creatrix of many a supersonic superfood tonic. Include all of the listed superfoods or whichever ones you prefer. Serve in wine or champagne glasses for a regal effect. This beverage will keep your guests going for hours on a natural high.

MAKES EIGHT 8-OUNCE SERVINGS

2 cups water

2 cups pineapple cubes

½ cup shredded coconut

¼ cup peeled and diced fresh ginger

2 tablespoons hemp seeds

4 cups ice

2 tablespoons to ¼ cup agave nectar, or to taste

1 teaspoon vanilla extract

Pinch of cayenne

1 (3½-ounce) package Sambazon açaí
(optional) (see Tips and Tricks)

2 tablespoons raw cacao powder (optional)

1 tablespoon maca powder
(optional) (see Tips and Tricks)

½ teaspoon spirulina (optional)

1. Combine the water, pineapple, coconut, ginger, and hemp seeds in a blender and blend until smooth. Pour through a cheesecloth or fine-mesh strainer into a 2-quart pitcher.
2. Combine in the blender the ice, agave, vanilla, cayenne, and whichever of the remaining ingredients you wish to include. Start blending, adding the pineapple mixture through the top as needed to blend until smooth. Pour into the pitcher and stir it up.

Tips and Tricks

Superfoods such as açaí and maca root powder are available at most health food stores. Açaí can be found frozen in individual serving packets. Maca root powder should be on the shelves with the other superfoods and supplements. If you don't see them, ask if you can place a special order.

LIVE SPRING ROLLS

Who doesn't love those salty deep-fried spring rolls dipped in that mysterious sugary, syrupy sauce served up at most Asian food restaurants? What's in those things, anyway? Well we certainly cannot answer that question, but we know what goes in to these delectable rolls: a rainbow assortment of all-natural whole foods and garden-fresh herbs. For extra fun and conversation starters, serve them Vietnamese style, with all of the fillings and the Swiss chard wrappers laid out on a plate for everyone to assemble to taste.

MAKES 8 ROLLS

4–8 Swiss chard or romaine lettuce leaves

½ cup grated carrot

½ cup grated beet

½ medium-size red bell pepper, seeded and sliced thinly

½ cup sprouts
(sunflower, clover, mung, or a combination)

8 large leaves fresh basil

4 sprigs fresh mint

Spring Roll Dipping Sauce

¾ cup raw tahini

½ cup water

2 tablespoons agave nectar

4 teaspoons Nama Shoyu

1 tablespoon freshly squeezed lemon juice

2 teaspoons peeled and grated fresh ginger

1. If the chard leaves are large, only use four, cut them in half, and remove the stems. If they are small, use all eight and leave most of the stem if it is pliable enough.
2. Lay out all of the spring roll fillings and wrappers on a plate or two. Whisk all of the dipping sauce ingredients together until fully combined. Serve immediately.

Variations

- Substitute raw almond butter for the tahini in the dipping sauce.
- Add or substitute different filling ingredients, such as green onion, diced jicama, thinly sliced chile peppers, red cabbage, or daikon. Mango or papaya slices would also jazz up the mixture.
- For a not-so-raw variation, add bean thread or rice stick noodles to the fillings.

Holiday Feast

This suggested menu is great for Thanksgiving. For a spring or summer feast, you may want to put together something a bit lighter, such Live Mango Gazpacho (page 153), Greek Salad (page 144), Macadamia Nut–Crusted Tofu (page 224), Southwest Roasted Asparagus and Corn (page 179), and Live Chocolate Mousse (page 254).

> Spinach–Herb Stuffed Portobellos (page 204)
> Roasted Garlic Mashed Potatoes (page 235)
> Tofu or Tempeh Cutlets (see page 27) with
>   Mushroom-Onion Gravy (page 236)
> Green Bean Almandine (recipe follows)
> Salad with Dressing (page 128)
> Holiday Nog (recipe follows)
> Baked Apple Crisp (page 271)

GREEN BEAN ALMANDINE

One of the ways we create an authentic feel to our vegan holiday meals is to include familiar dishes such as this. The green beans are a lovely addition, with their vibrant color—be sure not to overcook them. If green beans are unavailable, asparagus, zucchini, or even broccoli work as yummy replacements.

MAKES EIGHT ½-CUP SERVINGS

¼ cup almond slivers

1 cup water

1 pound fresh green beans, ends trimmed (about 4 cups)

3 tablespoons olive oil

2 tablespoons freshly squeezed lemon juice

2 teaspoons minced fresh garlic (optional)

2 tablespoons vegan butter (optional)

Sea salt and black pepper

1. Preheat the oven or a toaster oven to 350°F. Place the almonds on a baking sheet and bake until golden brown, about 3 minutes.
2. While the almonds are baking, place the water in a large sauté pan over medium-high heat. Bring to a boil, add the green beans, and cook until just tender, about 5 minutes, stirring frequently, ideally with a handy pair of tongs. Drain all excess water if any remains.
3. Add the oil, lemon juice, garlic, and vegan butter, if using, and gently toss well. Place in a casserole dish or on a serving platter. Top with the almonds and enjoy.

Variations
- Add 3 tablespoons of minced red bell pepper for color.
- Replace the almonds with pine nuts or pecans, raw or toasted (see page 26).
- You can also sauté the garlic in the oil and vegan butter. Add the almond slivers and cook for 1 minute, stirring frequently. Pour this over the cooked beans.

HOLIDAY NOG

This egg-free recipe makes a yummy sweet beverage available to you at all times, not just the holidays. For the creamiest nog, use Silk creamer.

MAKES 1 QUART

1 quart Silk creamer or vanilla soy milk

¼ cup pure maple syrup

1 teaspoon vanilla extract

½ teaspoon ground cinnamon

1 teaspoon ground nutmeg

½ teaspoon almond extract

2 tablespoons arrowroot powder

4 tablespoons cold water

1. Heat the soy creamer in a pot over medium heat. When it approaches boiling, lower the heat to a simmer. Whisk in all of the ingredients except the arrowroot and water.
2. Whisk the arrowroot and water together in a small bowl or measuring cup, and add to the pot. Whisk until the liquid thickens, about 5 minutes. Pour into glasses. Sprinkle with the cinnamon before serving. Happy Holiday!

Variation
- For those wishing for a thinner nog, use only 1 tablespoon of arrowroot dissolved in 2 tablespoons of cold water.

Acknowledgments

We would like to give thanks to our parents and to all of our friends and family who helped make this book possible. Thanks to Daniel Rhoda, for introducing us to our agent, Marilyn Allen of Allen O'Shea Literary Agency. Thank you, Marilyn, for your support and vision. Thanks to Matthew Lore of Da Capo Press, for believing in us and our concept.

A hearty thanks to Renee Sedlier, our rock-star editor, for her amazing contributions. Many thanks also to editor Cisca Schreefel and copy editor Iris Bass for their valuable input.

Give thanks to Bo and Star Rinaldi, for their eternal guidance, inspiration, and support.

Thanks to Jessyka Murray, for editing and proofreading. Thank you once again to our recipe developers and testers: Jessyka Murray, Elizabeth Warfield Murray, Lisa Parker, Gia Baiocchi, Roland Barker, Keli Ranke, Aaron Murray, Ryan Hughes, and Neil and Erica Greene.

Love and gratitude to Malana Fiore, for her assistance with the food styling.

Thanks to Dawn Reinfeld for the Hanalei Kitchen photos.

Special thanks to Deborah Madison, for her kind generosity in contributing the foreword. Deborah is a pioneer in the vegetarian movement and we are honored to have her participation in this book. You can visit her online at www.deborah madison.com.

METRIC CONVERSIONS

- The recipes in this book have not been tested with metric measurements, so some variations might occur.
- Remember that the weight of dry ingredients varies according to the volume or density factor: 1 cup of flour weighs far less than 1 cup of sugar, and 1 tablespoon doesn't necessarily hold 3 teaspoons.

— General Formulas for Metric Conversion

Ounces to grams	$\Rightarrow$ ounces × 28.35 = grams
Grams to ounces	$\Rightarrow$ grams × 0.035 = ounces
Pounds to grams	$\Rightarrow$ pounds × 453.5 = grams
Pounds to kilograms	$\Rightarrow$ pounds × 0.45 = kilograms
Cups to liters	$\Rightarrow$ cups × 0.24 = liters
Fahrenheit to Celsius	$\Rightarrow$ (°F – 32) × 5 ÷ 9 = °C
Celsius to Fahrenheit	$\Rightarrow$ (°C × 9) ÷ 5 + 32 = °F

— Linear Measurements

½ inch = 1½ cm
1 inch = 2½ cm
6 inches = 15 cm
8 inches = 20 cm
10 inches = 25 cm
12 inches = 30 cm
20 inches = 50 cm

— Volume (Dry) Measurements

¼ teaspoon = 1 milliliter
½ teaspoon = 2 milliliters
¾ teaspoon = 4 milliliters
1 teaspoon = 5 milliliters
1 tablespoon = 15 milliliters
¼ cup = 59 milliliters
⅓ cup = 79 milliliters
½ cup = 118 milliliters
⅔ cup = 158 milliliters
¾ cup = 177 milliliters
1 cup = 225 milliliters
4 cups or 1 quart = 1 liter
½ gallon = 2 liters
1 gallon = 4 liters

— Volume (Liquid) Measurements

1 teaspoon = ⅙ fluid ounce = 5 milliliters
1 tablespoon = ½ fluid ounce = 15 milliliters
2 tablespoons = 1 fluid ounce = 30 milliliters
¼ cup = 2 fluid ounces = 60 milliliters
⅓ cup = 2⅔ fluid ounces = 79 milliliters
½ cup = 4 fluid ounces = 118 milliliters
1 cup or ½ pint = 8 fluid ounces = 250 milliliters
2 cups or 1 pint = 16 fluid ounces = 500 milliliters
4 cups or 1 quart = 32 fluid ounces = 1,000 milliliters
1 gallon = 4 liters

— Oven Temperature Equivalents, Fahrenheit (F) and Celsius (C)

100°F = 38°C
200°F = 95°C
250°F = 120°C
300°F = 150°C
350°F = 180°C
400°F = 205°C
450°F = 230°C

— Weight (Mass) Measurements

1 ounce = 30 grams
2 ounces = 55 grams
3 ounces = 85 grams
4 ounces = ¼ pound = 125 grams
8 ounces = ½ pound = 240 grams
12 ounces = ¾ pound = 375 grams
16 ounces = 1 pound = 454 grams

Appendix A: Supplemental Information

Nothing will benefit human health and increase
the chances for survival of life on Earth
as much as the evolution to a vegetarian diet.
—ALBERT EINSTEIN

Why Vegan?

A vegetarian diet is one that does not include meat, fish, or poultry. There are three types of vegetarian diets. A "lacto-ovo vegetarian" diet includes eggs and dairy products. A "lacto-vegetarian" diet includes dairy products, but not eggs. "Vegan" is used to describe a diet and lifestyle that does not include the use or consumption of animal based products. This means vegans also avoid wearing leather and silk, and products tested on animals. The phrase "plant-based" is often used instead of the word "vegan."

Far from being a fad diet, there is a rich history of vegetarianism dating back to the ancient Brahmin priestly class in India. It is reputed that Pythagoras, the famous ancient Greek philosopher and mathematician, brought Brahmin knowledge to the West after traveling to India. Since then, countless visionaries, deep thinkers, and healers have adopted this form of diet. Today we find many celebrities, models, world-class athletes, body builders, physical trainers, physicians, and everyday folks have turned to vegetarianism as a way of life.

All have their own reasons for including plant-based foods in their diet. A majority do so for health reasons and the positive benefits they experience, such as

315

weight loss and increased energy. Others do so as an effort to conserve the earth's limited resources. Some restrain from eating animal products for moral, ethical, or religious reasons.

Optimal Health

There is somewhat of a revolution occurring in the medical world, surrounding the benefits of a plant-based diet. Renowned doctors such as Dr. Caldwell Esselstyn Jr. and Dr. Dean Ornish have successfully reversed instances of heart disease with programs that incorporate vegan foods. Dr. John McDougall and Dr. Gabriel Cousens have likewise had success reversing certain forms of diabetes.

The evidence continues to mount that overconsumption of the saturated fat and cholesterol in animal products leads to serious health problems, such as obesity, heart disease, diabetes, hypertension, gout, kidney stones, and certain forms of cancer.

In addition, animals raised on factory farms are routinely given hormones to accelerate their rate of growth for maximum profit. Antibiotics are used to protect their health as they are housed and transported in less than sanitary conditions. These drugs inevitably make their way into the bodies of the humans that consume them.

In their 1995 report, the U.S. Department of Agriculture and the U.S. Department of Health and Human Services affirmed that all of the body's nutritional needs can be met through a well-planned plant-based diet. The American Dietetic Association and Dieticians of Canada likewise state that "well-planned vegan and other types of vegetarian diets are appropriate for all stages of the life cycle, including during pregnancy, lactation, infancy, childhood and adolescence."

May this forever dispel the myth that a vegan diet is nutritionally lacking in any way. For all concerned parents, rest assured that a vegan diet provides all of the protein, calcium, iron, and all other vital nutrients needed for us to thrive.

Preserving the Environment

We live on a beautiful planet with a limited amount of resources. Fortunately, now more than ever there is public awareness regarding "going green" to preserve our environmental heritage for future generations. Earth Day celebrations, rainforest preservation, and global warming initiatives are becoming more widespread.

What is less known is that adopting a plant-based diet is considered by many to be the single most effective step we can take to protect our environment.

World scientists agree that global warming poses a serious risk to humanity and life as we know it. The key to reducing global warming is to reduce activities that produce the greenhouse gases that cause the earth's temperature to rise. According to a 2006 UN Report "Livestock's Long Shadow," raising livestock for food consumption is responsible for 18 percent of all greenhouse gases emitted. That's more than the entire world's transportation industry combined!

In fact, the overall environmental impact of a plant-based diet is a fraction of that of a meat based one. Here are some talking points for your next cocktail party:

- The livestock population of the United States consumes enough grain and soybeans each year to feed over five times the human population of the country. Animals are fed over 80 percent of the corn and 95 percent of the oats that are grown on our soil.
- Less than half of the harvested agricultural acreage goes to feed people.
- According to the USDA, one acre of land can produce 20,000 pounds of vegetables. This same amount of land can only produce 165 pounds of meat.
- It takes sixteen pounds of grain to produce one pound of meat.
- It requires 3½ acres of land per person to support a meat centered diet, 1½ acres of land to support a lacto-ovo vegetarian diet, and ⅙ of an acre of land to support a plant-based diet.
- If Americans were to reduce meat consumption by just 10 percent, it would free up 12 million tons of grain annually.
- Half of the water used in the United States goes to irrigate land growing feed and fodder for livestock. It takes approximately 2,500 gallons of water to produce a single pound of meat. Similarly, it takes approximately 4,000 gallons of water to provide a day's worth of food per person for a meat-centered diet, 1,200 gallons for a lacto-ovo vegetarian diet, and 300 gallons for a plant-based diet.
- Developing nations use land to raise beef for wealthier nations instead of utilizing that land for sustainable agriculture practices.
- Topsoil is the dark, rich soil that supplies the nutrients to the food we grow. It takes five hundred years to produce an inch of topsoil. This topsoil is rapidly vanishing due to clear-cutting of forests and cattle-grazing practices.

- For each acre of forestland cleared for human purposes, seven acres of forest is cleared for grazing livestock or growing livestock feed. This includes federal land that is leased for cattle-grazing purposes. This policy greatly accelerates the destruction of our precious forests.
- To support cattle grazing, South and Central America are destroying their rainforests. These rainforests contain close to half of all the species on Earth and many medicinal plants. Over a thousand species a year are becoming extinct and most of these are from rainforest and tropical settings. This practice also causes the displacement of indigenous peoples who have been living in these environments for countless generations.
- The factory farm industry is one of the largest polluters of our groundwater due to the chemicals, pesticides, and run-off waste that is inherent in its practices.
- Over 60 million people die of starvation every year. This means that we are feeding grain to animals while our fellow humans are dying of starvation in mind staggering numbers.

For those concerned about our environment, it all boils down to the question of sustainability. What is the most sustainable way for us to feed and support the growing human population? In the news we hear a lot about food shortages, about protests and riots over the rising cost of food. When you look at the disproportionate amount of land, water, and resources it takes to support a meat-based diet, it makes a lot of sense for us to introduce more plant-based foods into our way of life. Whether by going completely vegan or simply including more vegan meals each week, every little bit helps.

Much of this environmental information is provided by John Robbins, a pioneer in the promotion of the health and environmental benefits of a plant-based lifestyle. He is the author of the landmark *Diet for a New America*. His latest work, *Healthy at 100*, is a must-read in-depth exploration of health and longevity. He also founded EarthSave International to educate, inspire, and empower people around the world.

It's Cool to Be Kind

Many people adopt a vegetarian diet because of religious or moral beliefs that prohibit the killing of animals. These folks feel we are meant to be stewards and caretakers of the earth and its inhabitants and do not wish to support practices that inflict suffering on any creature that has the capacity to feel pain.

The small family farm where husbandry practices engendered a certain respect for the animals that were used for food is becoming a thing of the past. Today, most of the world's meat, dairy, and egg production occurs on massive factory farms that are owned by agribusiness conglomerates. This has brought about practices that view the raising and transportation of farm animals solely in terms of their ability to generate profits.

Animals are routinely given chemicals and antibiotics to keep them alive in these conditions. To increase the weight of cows, many are fed sawdust, plastic, tallow, grease, and cement dust seasoned with artificial flavors and aromas. Mother pigs on factory farms are kept in crates that are so small they are unable to turn around. Dairy cows are forced to remain pregnant most of their lives and are injected with hormones to increase milk production. Male calves born from these cows are often raised to become "veal." This practice consists of confining a newborn calf to a crate that is so small that he is unable to turn around. This is to ensure that the flesh remains tender. They are fed diets that are deliberately iron deficient, a practice that induces anemia and allows the flesh to remain white. After four months or so in these conditions, the calf is slaughtered to produce "veal."

Go Organic

The Organic Trade Association states that "organic farming is based on practices that maintain soil fertility, while assisting nature's balance through diversity and recycling of energy and nutrients. This method also strives to avoid or reduce the use of synthetic fertilizers and pest controls. Organic foods are processed, packaged, transported and stored to retain maximum nutritional value, without the use of artificial preservatives, coloring or other additives, irradiation or synthetic pesticides."

Some people wonder if it's worth it to buy organic. To that we reply that many of the chemicals in commercial pesticides and fertilizers have not been tested for their long-term effects on humans. Is it worth it to take that chance with your health and the health of your family? Organically grown foods represent a cycle of sustainability that improves topsoil fertility, enhances nutrition, and ensures food security.

Organic farmers employ farming methods that respect the fragile balance of our ecosystem. This results in a fraction of the groundwater pollution and topsoil depletion generated by conventional methods. Most people have also found the taste and nutrient quality of organic products superior to that of conventionally grown food.

Purchasing local, seasonal, and organically grown food is also an extremely effective way to reduce your environmental impact. Buying local saves the huge amount of energy it takes to transport food—sometimes across oceans and continents.

Another reason to support organic farmers has to do with the health of the farm workers themselves. Farm workers on conventional farms are exposed to high levels of toxic pesticides on a daily basis. Organic farm workers don't have to encounter these risks.

Lastly, by supporting organic farmers, we are supporting small, family farms. This once prevalent method of farming is rapidly disappearing. This is due to the small farmer's inability to compete with the heavily subsidized agribusiness farms that use synthetic soil, pesticides, crop dusters, and heavy machinery on lands that encompass thousands of acres.

For more information on organic farming, visit your local farmers' market and talk to the farmers. You can also check out the Web sites for the International Federation of Organic Agriculture Movements, the Organic Consumers Association, and the Organic Trade Association listed in appendix B.

GMO Alert

A GMO (genetically engineered and modified organism) is a plant, animal, or microorganism that has had its genetic code altered—typically by introducing genes from another organism. This process gives the GMO food characteristics that are not present in its original form. Many feel this practice goes against nature and poses a profound threat to people, the environment, and our agricultural heritage.

GMO seed manufacturers maintain that this makes the seed more pest resistant, promotes higher yields, or enhances nutrition. The fact is that the long-term effects of these seeds on the consumer and our genetic pool is still unknown. We believe this untested engineering might be dangerous to human health in the long term. By definition, eating organic foods eliminates GMOs from our food supply.

There are even GMO seeds that are referred to as assassin seeds. The plant that grows from these seeds produces seeds that are infertile. This prevents the replication of the genetic bond. This means that farmers must constantly purchase seeds every year from the companies that manufacture them.

Many communities around the world have succeeded in becoming GMO-free. Please join us in this critical movement to move our agriculture away from genetic engineering and toward truly sustainable agriculture. For more information, you may visit the Non-GMO Project at www.nongmoproject.org.

Composting: The Cycle of Life

Composting is the method of breaking down food waste, grass trimmings, and leaves to create nutrient-rich and fertile soil. It's the next step we can take toward creating a more sustainable method of growing our food. Compost contains nitrogen and micronutrients to keep the soil healthy and can be used as a mulch and soil amendment. When the soil is healthy, plant yields are higher, and fertilizers and pesticides aren't as necessary.

Composting completes the cycle of life from seed to table and back to the earth. Many communities sponsor composting programs and can give you all the tools and instructions you need to succeed. Check out www.compostguide.com for a complete guide to composting.

Appendix B: Resource Guide

In this section we provide our recommendations for you to explore the subject matter in the book more in depth. Follow these leads for a lifetime of exploration into the art of healthy living.

Further Reading

Bailey, Steven, and Larry Trivieri, Jr. *Juice Alive: The Ultimate Guide to Juicing Remedies.* Garden City Park, NY: Square One Publishers, 2006.

Brazier, Brendan. *The Thrive Diet: The Whole Food Way to Lose Weight, Reduce Stress, and Stay Healthy for Life.* New York: Da Capo Press, 2007.

Campbell, T. Colin, and Thomas M. Campbell II. *The China Study: The Most Comprehensive Study of Nutrition Ever Conducted and the Startling Implications for Diet, Weight Loss, and Long-Term Health.* Dallas, TX: Benbella Books, 2006.

Cousens, Gabriel. *Conscious Eating.* Berkeley, CA: North Atlantic Books, 2000.

_____. *Rainbow Green Live-Food Cuisine.* Berkeley, CA: North Atlantic Books, 2003.

Esselstyn, Caldwell. *Prevent and Reverse Heart Disease.* New York: Avery Publishing, 2007.

Fuhrman, Joel, M.D. *Eat to Live: The Revolutionary Formula for Fast and Sustained Weight Loss.* Boston, MA: Little, Brown, and Company, 2005.

Graham, Dr. Douglas N. *The 80/10/10 Diet.* Key Largo, FL: FoodnSport Press, 2006.

Jacobson, Michael, Ph.D. *Six Arguments for a Greener Diet: How a Plant-Based Diet Could Save Your Health and the Environment.* Washington, D.C.: Center for Science in the Public Interest, 2006.

Kulvinskas, Viktoras. *Survival into the 21st Century: Planetary Healers Manual*. Woodstock Valley, CT: 21st Century Publications, 1981.

Lyman, Howard. *Mad Cowboy: Plain Truth from the Cattle Rancher Who Won't Eat Meat*. New York: Scribner, 2001.

Marcus, Erik. *Vegan: The New Ethics of Eating*. Ithaca, NY: McBooks Press, 2001.

Meyerowitz, Steve. *Sprouts, the Miracle Food: The Complete Guide to Sprouting*. Great Barrington, MA: Sproutman Publications, 1999.

Monarch, Matthew. *Raw Success*. Ojai, CA: Matthew Monarch, 2007.

Ornish, Dean. *Dr. Dean Ornish's Program for Reversing Heart Disease: The Only System Scientifically Proven to Reverse Heart Disease Without Drugs or Surgery*. New York: Ivy Books, 1995.

Pitchford, P. *Healing with Whole Foods*. Berkeley, CA: North Atlantic Books, 1993.

Reinfeld, Mark, and Bo Rinaldi. *Vegan Fusion World Cuisine: Extraordinary Recipes and Timeless Wisdom from the Celebrated Blossoming Lotus Restaurants*. New York: Beaufort Books, 2007.

Reinfeld, Mark, Bo Rinaldi, and Jennifer Murray. *The Complete Idiot's Guide to Eating Raw*. Indianapolis, IN: Alpha Books, 2008.

Robbins, John. *Diet for a New America*. Tiburon, CA: HJ Kramer, 1987.

_____. *Healthy at 100*. New York: Random House, 2006.

Stuart, Tristram. *The Bloodless Revolution: A Cultural History of Vegetarianism from 1600 to Modern Times*. New York: W. W. Norton, 2007.

Tuttle, Will, Ph.D. *World Peace Diet: Eating for Spiritual Health and Social Harmony*. Brooklyn, NY: Lantern Books, 2005.

Walker, Dr. Norman. *Fresh Vegetable and Fruit Juices: What's Missing in Your Body?* Revised Edition. Prescott, AZ: Norwalk Press, 1981.

Wigmore, Ann. *The Hippocrates Diet and Health Program*. New York: Avery Publishing, 1983.

Wolfe, David. *The Sunfood Diet Success System*, 6th ed. San Diego, CA: Maul Brothers Publishing, 2006.

Online Resources

So many Web sites and blogs promote a vegan and sustainable way of life. You can also join vegan groups on social networking sites such as MySpace and Facebook. Do a search for such key words as *vegan*, *organic*, and *sustainable*, and countless sites will come up. Here are some of our favorites.

Vegan & Veg-Friendly Web sites

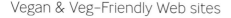

www.veganfusion.com
This is our Web site, which contains links to the informative Vegan Fusion Newsletter. Be sure to sign up to receive free recipes, inspiration, and the latest current events.

www.earthsave.org
Founded by John Robbins, EarthSave is doing what it can to promote a shift to a plant-based diet. It posts news, information, and resources, and publishes a magazine.

www.happycow.net
Happy Cow is a searchable dining guide to vegetarian restaurants, natural health food stores, information on vegetarian nutrition, raw foods, and vegan recipes.

www.peta.org
People for the Ethical Treatment of Animals (PETA), the largest animal rights organization in the world, is dedicated to establishing and protecting the rights of all animals.

www.animalconcerns.org
Animal Concerns Community serves as a clearinghouse for information on the Internet related to animal rights and welfare.

www.aspca.org
The American Society for the Prevention of Cruelty to Animals (ASPCA) provides effective means to prevent animal cruelty in the United States.

www.farmusa.org
Farm Animal Reform Movement (FARM) is an organization advocating a plant-based diet and humane treatment of farm animals through grassroots programs.

www.hsus.org
The Humane Society of the United States (HSUS) wishes to create a world where humans relate to animals with compassion.

www.vegweb.com
A vegetarian megasite with recipes, photos, articles, an online store, and more.

www.godairyfree.org
Go Dairy Free is a comprehensive Web site with information on how to cook, shop, and dine dairy-free, while still promoting a healthy lifestyle.

www.compassionatecooks.com
Compassionate Cooks offers vegetarian cooking classes, cooking videos, and recipes.

www.tastyandmeatless.com
Tasty and Meatless is a weekly vegetarian television series on Time Warner Cable.

www.vegtv.com
The site for Veg TV video production company, producing and streaming original content about vegetarian and vegan food, health, nutrition, and eco-travel.

www.vegsoc.org
The Vegetarian Society is a registered charity committed to promoting the health, environmental, and animal welfare benefits of a vegetarian diet.

www.vegan.com
The popular site of Erik Marcus, geared toward the aspiring and long-term vegan that features articles, interviews, product evaluations, book reviews, and more.

www.vegan.org
Vegan Action is a nonprofit grassroots organization dedicated to educating people about the many benefits of a vegan lifestyle.

www.veganpassions.com
Vegan Passions is a free online dating site for meeting single vegans.

www.vrg.org
The Vegetarian Resource Group (VRG) is a nonprofit organization dedicated to educating the public on vegetarianism, including information on health, nutrition, ecology, ethics, and world hunger.

www.vegdining.com
A vegetarian dining guide that includes an international search option, a monthly veggie restaurant contest, and the opportunity to purchase a VegDining card for discounts at participating veggie restaurants.

www.thevegetariansite.com
An extensive online source for vegan and vegetarian living, including health and nutrition info, animal rights info, news, and complete online shopping.

www.vegan.meetup.com
Meet up with other vegans in your town!

www.veganpeace.com
Vegan Peace is striving toward peacefully sharing our Earth and includes information about veganism, animal cruelty, recipes, cookbook reviews, and nutritional information.

www.keepkidshealthy.com
A guide for raising vegan children, with advice on providing your child with an early start toward leading a long and healthy life.

www.vegnews.com

An award-winning magazine that focuses on a vegetarian lifestyle, featuring news, events, recipes, book reviews, the best veg products, travel tales, interviews, celebrity buzz, and more.

www.veganfitness.net

Vegan Fitness is a community-driven message board that seeks to provide a supportive, educational, and friendly environment for vegans, vegetarians, and those seeking to go vegan.

www.vegansociety.com

The Vegan Society promotes ways of living free of animal products for the benefit of people, animals and the environment.

www.veganpet.com.au

Veganpet provides nutritionally complete and balanced pet food and information on raising vegan pets.

www.vegfamily.com

Comprehensive resource for raising vegan children, including pregnancy, vegan recipes, book reviews, product reviews, message board, and more.

www.vegcooking.com

Features hundreds of vegetarian and vegan recipes with spotlights on vegetarian and vegan foods, products, menus, and restaurants.

www.veganbodybuilding.com

Vegan Body Building and Fitness is the Web site of vegan body builder Robert Cheeke and features articles, videos, products, and a forum for the active vegan.

www.vegsource.com

Features over 10,000 vegetarian and vegan recipes, discussion boards, nutritionists, medical doctors, experts, authors, articles, newsletter, and the vegetarian community.

www.pcrm.org

The Physicians Committee for Responsible Medicine (PCRM) is a nonprofit organization that promotes preventive medicine, conducts clinical research, and encourages higher standards for ethics and effectiveness in research.

www.ivu.org

The World Union of Vegetarian/ Vegan Societies has been promoting vegetarianism worldwide since 1908.

www.vegetarianteen.com

An online magazine with articles on vegetarian teen lifestyle, activism, nutrition, social issues, and more.

Organic & Gardening Web sites

www.ota.com

The Organic Trade Association Web site will tell you anything you want to know about the term *organic*, from food to textiles to health-care products. The OTA's mission is to encourage global sustainability through promoting and protecting the growth of diverse organic trade.

www.ifoam.org

International Federation of Organic Agriculture Movements is the umbrella organization for hundreds of organic organizations worldwide.

www.organicconsumers.org

The Organic Consumers Association is an online, grassroots, nonprofit organization dealing with issues of food safety, industrial agriculture, genetic engineering, corporate accountability, and environmental sustainability.

www.seedsofchange.com

This site is now divided in two sections—one is for seeds and gardening, the other is their online store of organic food products.

www.permacultureactivist.net

The Permaculture Activist reports the work of grassroots landscape designers and social change artists from around the world.

www.organicgardening.com

Find out where to get your soil tested, manage pests without using chemicals, and read vegetable- and flower-growing guides.

www.avant-gardening.com

A site advocating organic gardening with information on composting, soil building, permaculture principles, botany, companion and intensive planting, and more.

www.wwoof.org

World-Wide Opportunities on Organic Farms (WWOOF) is an association helping those who wish to volunteer on organic farms internationally.

www.gefoodalert.org

GE Food Alert Campaign Center is a coalition of seven organizations committed to testing and labeling genetically engineered food.

www.earthflow.com

Earthflow is an all natural approach to permaculture design, offering garden tours and training programs, including permaculture courses.

www.biodynamics.com

The Biodynamic Farming and Gardening Association supports and promotes biodynamic farming, the oldest nonchemical agricultural movement.

Environmental & Sustainability Web sites

www.conservation.org

Conservation International is involved in many conservation projects worldwide. On their site you can calculate your carbon footprint based on your living situation, car, travel habits, and diet.

www.greenpeace.org

Greenpeace focuses on the most crucial worldwide threats to our planet's biodiversity and environment.

www.nrdcwildplaces.org

Natural Resources Defense Council (NRDC) is an environmental action group with over one million members working to safeguard the American continents' natural systems.

www.dinegreen.com

The Green Restaurant Association (GRA) is a national nonprofit organization that provides a convenient way for all sectors of the restaurant industry, which represents 10 percent of the U.S. economy, to become more environmentally sustainable.

www.sierraclub.org

The Sierra Club is America's oldest, largest, and most influential grassroots environmental organization.

www.pirg.org

The Public Interest Research Group (PIRG) is an alliance of state-based, citizen-funded organizations that provide result-oriented activism to protect the environment, develop a fair marketplace, and encourage a responsive, democratic government. Look for your state's PIRG on their Web site.

www.higean.org/kauai

GMO-Free Kauai is a grassroots organization created to raise awareness and educate the public about the health, economic, and environmental risks of genetically engineered and modified organisms. Hawaii, including Kauai, is one of the top two states in the country for open-air GMO field testing.

www.ran.org

Rainforest Action Network is working to protect tropical rainforests around the world and the human rights of those living in and around those forests.

www.childrenoftheearth.org

Children of the Earth United is a children's environmental education Web site that educates the public on ecological concepts and aims to provide a forum for people to share knowledge and ideas.

Eco-Friendly Products & Services

www.veganessentials.com

Vegan Essentials is the place to shop for vegan clothes, shoes, cosmetics, and so much more.

www.foodfightgrocery.com

Food Fight! Grocery is an all-vegan convenience store located in Portland, Oregon, with an online market that emphasizes junk foods, imports, and fun stuff.

www.goldminenaturalfood.com

An online source for a vast selection of organic foods, raw foods, macrobiotic, vegan, gluten-free, Asian, gourmet, and specialty foods, as well as natural cookware and home products.

www.gaiam.com

Gaiam is the premier source for sustainable green living and fitness lifestyle products.

www.VoiceYourself.com

A nonprofit started by Woody Harrelson and his wife, Laura Louie, to encourage citizens to protect the quality of our air, soil, and water through everyday choices and actions.

www.vitamix.com

Find the latest Vita-Mix blenders here on the official site, including factory-reconditioned models that still come with a seven-year warranty. For free shipping in the continental United States, enter code 06–002510.

www.877juicer.com

This Web site carries way more than juicers, including everything kitchen related, plus air purifiers, books, and articles.

www.sproutpeople.com

Sprout People provides for all of your sprouting needs, including seeds, sprouting jars, lids, mesh screens, canning rings, and advice to the beginner or advanced sprouters.

www.excaliburdehydrator.com

Get your dehydrator right from the manufacturer, where parts and accessories are also available.

www.pureprescriptions.com

Pure prescriptions is an online superstore for high quality nutritional products, complete with free consultations and a health library.

www.OrganicAvenue.com

Organic Avenue provides tactical support for the naturalist lifestyle, featuring a full online store offering natural fiber fashion, housewares, accessories, and much more.

www.greenpeople.org

Green People provides a directory of eco-friendly products and services.

www.ecoproducts.com

Ecoproducts is the premier site for biodegradable and compostable food service products and environmentally friendly household supplies.

Raw Food Lifestyle Web sites

www.sunfood.com

David Wolfe's Web site, Nature's First Law, provides the raw foodist with everything from food and supplements to appliances to books and personals ads.

www.goneraw.com

Gone Raw is a Web site created to help people share and discuss raw and vegan recipes from around the world.

www.rawfoods.com

Living and Raw Foods is the largest raw online community, with appliances for the raw foodist, chat rooms, blogs, articles, classifieds ads, and recipes.

www.gliving.tv

The G Living Network is a hip and modern green lifestyle network with videos and articles on living in an earth-friendly way, including raw recipes, sustainable fashion, technology, and household design.

www.brendanbrazier.com

Brendan Brazier is an Ironman Triathlete, speaker, and author of *The Thrive Diet.* You can find his book and his calendar of events here on this Web site.

www.highvibe.com

This site offers an online store, recipes, fasting information, testimonials, interviews, and much more.

www.rawfamily.com

On this Web site, Victoria Boutenko and her entire family share recipes and their secrets on life as a raw family.

www.living-foods.com

The largest online community dedicated to educating the world about the power of raw and live foods. This site is jam packed with information, classifieds, personals, books, and more.

Retreats & Workshops

www.treeoflife.nu

The Tree of Life Rejuvenation Center, located in Patagonia, Arizona, was started by raw food guru, Dr. Gabriel Cousens. The Center offers nightly rates, detox/cleansing packages, workshops, a live food café, apprenticeships, nutrition programs, and an online store.

www.drmcdougall.com

Dr. McDougall's Health and Medical Center in Santa Rosa, California, is like a first-class resort with health-sustaining benefits. The center offers ten-day programs as well as advanced programs for individuals interested in taking control of their own health.

www.rawfoodchef.com

The Living Light Culinary Arts Institute offers vegan raw food chef certification in a comprehensive seventeen-day program.

World Peace & Hunger Organizations

www.janegoodall.org

The Jane Goodall Institute celebrates the prospect of peace on Earth through a variety of initiatives and projects. A main focus is the Roots & Shoots Global Peace Initiative, which inspires youths to make the world a better place through project-based learning.

www.seva.org

The Seva Foundation offers programs that are developed in a way that builds self-reliance and are based on a vision of the connection between spirit, culture, and health.

www.worldpeacefoundation.org
World Peace Foundation seeks to advance the cause of peace through study, analysis, and the advocacy of wise action.

www.gandhi.ca
Mahatma Gandhi Canadian Foundation for World Peace Seeks to universally share knowledge of Mahatma Gandhi's beliefs and philosophies.

www.religioustolerance.org
Religious Tolerance is a megasite fostering peace among all nations and religions.

www.belief.net
The largest site on the Internet for pancultural religious tolerance, supporting a global vision for understanding and dispelling myths about faiths and beliefs.

www.foodnotbombs.net
Food Not Bombs is an all-volunteer organization that recovers food that would otherwise be thrown out and makes fresh hot vegetarian meals that are served in city parks, at peaceful protests, and other events to anyone without restriction.

www.thehungersite.com
The Hunger Site is a leader in online activism toward ending world hunger. With a click of your mouse button, an advertiser will make a donation to the cause. Visit often!

www.careusa.org
Care is one of the world's largest private international humanitarian organizations, whose goal is that every person enjoys at least the minimum standards required to live in dignity and security.

www.thp.org
The Hunger Project is an organization committed to end world hunger sustainably and through the empowerment of women.

www.worldhungeryear.org
World Hunger Year (WHY), founded by the late Harry Chapin, gets to the root causes of hunger and poverty by promoting grassroots, community-based solutions to create self-reliance, economic justice, and food security.

www.sacredsites.com
Places of Peace and Power: Sacred Sites and Pilgrimage Traditions of the World by anthropologist and photographer Martin Gray.

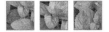

Glossary

Açaí the high antioxidant purple berry of the açaí palm, native to the Amazon. It's found mainly in frozen, dried, and freeze-dried forms as well as an ingredient in packaged smoothies and juices.

Agave nectar a sweetener from the agave cactus that ranges in color from golden to brown. Composed mainly of fructose and glucose, it has a low glycemic index and is about 1½ times sweeter than sugar.

Al dente an Italian phrase that describes pasta that's cooked until tender, but still firm with a slightly chewy texture.

Antioxidants disease fighting molecules that slow down or prevent the oxidation of other molecules by quenching damaging free radicals. Superfoods are rich in antioxidants.

Apple cider vinegar made from apples; look for the raw variety that preserves many of its nutrients and is considered to have beneficial healing qualities.

Arame a species of kelp high in calcium, protein, iron, iodine, and other vitamins and minerals.

Arrowroot a powdered starch made from the root of the arrowroot plant. Used as a thickener in sauces, soups, and desserts. Dissolve arrowroot with an equal amount of cold water before adding to the mixture being thickened.

Barley malt syrup a sweetener that is roughly half as sweet as honey or sugar. Made from sprouted barley, it has a nutty, caramel flavor.

Brown rice syrup a relatively neutral flavored sweetener made from cultured brown rice; it is roughly half as sweet as sugar.

Buckwheat a triangular-shaped seed often considered a grain. It's not related to wheat and is entirely gluten free. Raw groats are used in live food preparation. The roasted groat is called kasha.

Cacao beans the seeds of the cacao tree that are the source of chocolate. Cacao is the nutrient-rich, antioxidant power food of the Aztecs, Incans, and Mayans.

Capers peppercorn-size flower buds of a Mediterranean bush, capers are usually sun-dried and pickled in vinegar brine. They impart a tangy, salty flavor to dishes.

Carob a member of the legume family that is relatively high in protein. Also referred to as St. Johns Bread or Honey Locust, it may be used as an alternative to cocoa.

Celtic sea salt unrefined, with a high mineral content, this light gray salt is naturally harvested off the coast of France. It is one of the most highly regarded forms of salt.

Coconut butter a relatively new commercial product whereby the meat of mature coconuts is ground, like nut butters, into a creamy spread.

Coconut oil one of our favorite oils for high temperature heating. Although high in saturated fat, and therefore solid at room temperature, coconut oil is being studied for its healing potential.

Composting the natural biological process of breaking down food waste, grass trimmings, and leaves to create a nutrient-rich soil.

Culturing a simple process that introduces natural bacteria to a food to create delicacies such as plant-based cheeses, sauerkrauts, sour creams, and yogurts. These bacteria promote healthy flora in the digestive system and are known as probiotics.

Dehydrator a kitchen appliance used in live food preparation that removes water from food much like an oven but at much lower temperatures, thus preserving the food's nutrients, vitamins, and enzymes.

Dulse an iron-rich sea vegetable that is a good source of vitamin B6, fluoride, and potassium. Use the flakes as a salt replacement, sprinkled on salads, soups, or steamed veggies. The whole pieces make for a nutritious snack.

Flaxseeds small seeds packed with omega-3 essential fatty acids (EFAs) and other nutrients such as magnesium, phosphorus, and thiamin. They can be ground and used in baking to replace eggs. Their oil makes a fantastic, nutty salad dressing.

Free radicals atoms or molecules with unpaired electrons. Free-radical damage has been linked to the aging process.

Garbanzo beans also known as chickpeas, garbanzo beans are high in iron, folate, vitamin B6, magnesium, phosphorus, zinc, protein, and dietary fiber.

Goji berries also called the wolfberry, this small red fruit is well known in Asia for its antioxidant and nutrient content.

Hemp seeds these highly nutritious seeds from the Cannabis plant are a superior source of plant-based protein and essential fatty acids, are 100 percent legal, and do not contain any psychoactive properties.

Himalayan crystal salt considered one of the purest and least processed salts, it's more than 250 million years old, mined in the Himalayas by hand and carefully rinsed.

Jerusalem artichoke or "sunchoke" is the tuber of a plant from the sunflower family. It has a nutty, earthy flavor and many health benefits, including a good source of the soluble fiber inulin. It may be enjoyed grated raw in salads, steamed, or roasted in cubes.

Jicama a root vegetable grown and used widely in Mexico. Resembling a beet or a turnip, it can be small or quite large. Its skin is a beige color; the inside is white. The consistency is like a raw potato although the taste is sweet, like an apple.

Kaffir lime leaf the bay leaf of Southeast Asia, the kaffir lime leaf is added to stocks and soups and removed before serving. A must-have for all Thai dishes.

Kelp brown algae that grows in large, dense, underwater forests, some three stories high, in cold, clear waters. Growing as much as two feet per day, kelp is high in B vitamins, protein, iron, magnesium, and zinc and is a source of iodine.

Kombu a wide and flat seaweed, kombu is a good source of calcium, folate, and magnesium. We add it to beans while cooking to bring out the flavor of the bean and increase digestibility.

Lacto-ovo vegetarians vegetarians whose diet includes eggs and dairy products.

Lacto-vegetarians vegetarians whose diet includes dairy products but not eggs.

Lemongrass a grass popular in Thai and Vietnamese cuisine that imparts a citrus flavor and has been shown to possess antifungal properties.

Liquid Smoke purified water that has been infused with smoke. It adds a unique, smoky flavor to dishes. Only a small amount is necessary.

Live or living foods those raw foods that are soaked, sprouted, or cultured to enhance enzyme activity.

Maca a plant native to the mountainous regions of South America that is known to increase energy and endurance, this superfood contains fiber, protein, essential fats, and many essential minerals.

Maple syrup the boiled-down sap of sugar maple trees. It is rich in minerals such as manganese and zinc and contains fewer calories than honey. It is graded according to color and flavor. Grade A is the mildest and lightest, Grade C is the darkest and richest. Good for baking.

Mandoline a handy kitchen tool used to slice, julienne, or crinkle-cut harder vegetables quickly by hand.

Mirin a sweet and tangy Japanese rice cooking wine that many use as a "secret ingredient" to add a unique flavor to a variety of dishes.

Miso a salty paste made by fermenting soybeans, grains, and other beans. Used in many recipes, including dips, dressings, sauces, spreads, and the traditional soup. Boiling miso destroys many of its beneficial nutrients.

Molasses this syrup is a liquid by-product of the sugar refining process. It contains many of the nutrients of the sugar cane plant and has a strong, somewhat bitter-sweet flavor.

Nama Shoyu *nama* means "raw" or "unpasteurized"; *shoyu* is Japanese for "soy sauce." Nama Shoyu is an unpasteurized condiment made from cultured soybeans and wheat.

Nori a highly nutritious red algae that's shredded, dried, and pressed like paper, providing calcium, iron, and other vitamins and minerals

Nutritional yeast a plant-based culture consisting of up to 50 percent protein. The Red Star variety is a source of B vitamins including B12, naturally low in sodium and fat, and generally extracted from molasses. In cooking it is used to create a cheeselike flavor and is a favorite to sprinkle on salads, popcorn, and steamed vegetables.

Olive oil ranges in flavor from mild to strong. We recommend the organic extra-virgin cold-pressed variety, which is from the first pressing of the olives.

Organic farming a natural and environmentally friendly way to grow food without the use of chemical fertilizers and pesticides. Organic methods include, but are not limited to, crop rotation, integrated pest management, natural fertilizers, and composting.

Protein an important component of cells, tissues, organs, muscles, and bones. The current dietary guidelines recommend that healthy persons ingest 0.8 g daily per kg of body weight.

Quinoa an ancient Incan grain that is one of the highest plant sources of protein. It's also a source of calcium, iron, phosphorus, B vitamins, and vitamin E.

Raw foods foods that have not been cooked above a certain temperature, generally considered 116°F. See *Live or living foods*.

Rejuvelac this fermented beverage is high in friendly digestive bacteria. It is the strained-off soak water used when sprouting certain grains such as wheat and rye berries.

Roux a French term that describes a mixture of flour and oil, typically in a one-to-one ratio, which is used to thicken sauces, gravies, and soups.

Saffron the handpicked stigma or the saffron crocus flower, it's the most precious and expensive spice in the world. It imparts a bright orange-yellow color and an exotic flavor and aroma.

Sea salt made from evaporated sea water. Higher in minerals than commercially processed table salt. See also *Celtic sea salt*, and *Himalayan crystal salt*.

Seitan originating in ancient China, is sometimes referred to as "meat of wheat" or "Buddha food." It is wheat gluten dough that has been cooked in a broth with different types of seasonings.

Shoyu a traditional Japanese soy sauce that is made from fermented soy beans and wheat. It imparts a strong salty flavor. See also *Soy sauce* and *Tamari*.

Soy sauce a traditional Japanese condiment that is made from fermented soy beans and wheat. It imparts a strong salty flavor. See also *Shoyu* and *Tamari*.

Spelt a highly nutritious and ancient grain that is in the wheat family. It has a slightly nutty flavor and may be used to replace whole wheat flour in baked goods and pastas.

Spiralizer a kitchen tool that slices and shreds and allows you to create unique garnishes and continuous strands of "pasta" from vegetables such as zucchini or summer squash.

Spirulina a freshwater, blue-green algae containing protein, beta carotene, fatty acids, most B vitamins, as well as vitamins C, D, and E. Try this superfood in live pie fillings and crusts, smoothies, or sprinkled on salads and popcorn.

Sprouting the process of germination and growth that occurs after soaking and rinsing seeds. Sprouting greatly enhances a seed's nutritional profile.

Stevia leaf a member of the mint family originating in Paraguay, South America. Stevia is hundreds of times sweeter than sugar and is actually purported to benefit tooth health. For baking conversions, please visit www.steviashop.com/additional uses.php.

Sucanat abbreviation for "sugar cane natural"; a granular sweetener that consists of evaporated sugar cane juice. It has approximately the same sweetness as sugar but retains most of the vitamins and minerals of the sugar cane.

Superfoods nutrient-dense foods containing antioxidants. They promote optimal health and contain phytonutrients, vitamins, and minerals.

Tahini a paste made from finely ground sesame seeds, used in Middle Eastern and Mediterranean cooking. Tahini imparts a creamy, buttery flavor to dishes.

Tamari a traditional Japanese wheat-free soy sauce made from fermented soy beans that imparts a strong salty flavor. See also *Shoyu* and *Soy sauce*.

Tamarind a tropical fruit widely used in drinks, sauces, and pad thai. The pulp has a sweet and sour flavor and is rich in B vitamins and calcium. It's popular in chutney in Indian cuisine and is used in drinks around the world.

Tempeh originally from Indonesia, tempeh consists of soy beans cultured in a rice culture, then cooked. Many different varieties are created by mixing the soy bean with grains such as millet, wheat, or rice.

Tofu processed soy bean curd with origins in ancient China. It is commercially sold in a number of different forms including extra-firm, firm, soft, and silken. Each different form lends itself to a particular type of food preparation.

Turbinado sugar a large crystal created as a by-product from the first pressing of sugar cane. Moister than refined sugar, it is roughly equally as sweet as brown sugar and retains some molasses content.

Transition foods products or ingredients that assist us in switching from less healthful foods to healthier alternatives. Although not necessarily the most healthful items themselves, they fill a role in satisfying cravings. It's not recommended to have these transition foods make up a large part of our diet.

Umeboshi plum a Japanese plum that's salted, pickled, and aged for many years. The paste imparts a tangy, salty flavor to many dishes and is also used as a spread in nori rolls.

Wakame part of the kelp family, this green seaweed is popular in Asia and is used in soups, salads, and noodle dishes. It's high in calcium, niacin, thiamine, and B vitamins.

Wasabi powder a ground horseradish root that's pungent, and quite spicy. When combined with water, it forms a paste that is a traditional Japanese condiment.

Wheatgrass the grass grown from the wheat berry that's generally pressed into juice. Wheatgrass juice is a nutritional powerhouse that revitalizes, detoxifies, and cleanses the body.

Yakon this tuber is a distant relative of the sunflower. From the Andean region of South America, mineral rich yakon syrup has a dark brown color and is used as a low-calorie sweetener.

Index